ABCs of FITNESS

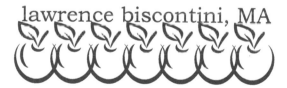

lawrence biscontini, MA

findLawrence.com

This book is printed on 60% post-consumer recycled paper as part of an environmentally-conscious decision to play part in the greening of the planet.

Fifth Edition

The ABC's of Fitness: An Alphabet Book to Wellness
© 2007 by Lawrence Biscontini, MA

Printed in the United States of America

Library of Congress Catalog Card Number:
ISBN 978-0-6151-4167-1

Published by:
FG2000 and Lulu.com

DEDICATION

On a personal scale, I dedicate this to Mother Barbara because I wrote it as if speaking to her in language she can understand <u>and use</u>. On a larger scale, I dedicate this to the people who—through no fault of their own—are so confused by contradictory information in the media about what simple steps they can take to make their lives better. These ABCs are for you.

GRATITUDE:

I humbly thank God for infinite blessings, inspiration, and energy, and Constance Mary Towers, the apotheosis of impromptu grace and elocution (for her unending understanding, eloquence, and positivism). She truly is covered with the fingerprints of God. I also thank Alana (for the "support and Scrabbles"); Maria Gavin; Sara Kooperman (this is your IDEA 'shout out'); Petra Kolber (for the professional advice); C Mark Rees (for FG2000), the entire Golden Door Puerto Rico team (for constant support both at my position and away from it), Stephanie Montgomery at Reebok, AFAA (especially Kim, Laurie and Lisa), ACE (especially Stacey, Kristie, and Brian), AEA (Julie and Angie), the AFPP (especially Tina Juan, Shirley, and Bam!), Mike and Stephanie Morris (for the teamwork on the BALL), Len Kravitz (for the mentoring and research); the gals at John and Ankie's Bodywork Gym in Mykonos; Rosi Manrara at AA for sending me off always so well; Laimi Largent, Diane Berson and J Sklar (for the details); Susan L. Fischer (for transcendence in education), Tom Snow (for the original "Yo-Ch" music), Robert Milazzo (for the photos); the Xerox Queen herself, Maria Kalofolia (for the truest friendship); Ankie and John (for the Bodywork Gym membership); Kathie and Peter Davis for IDEA; Maureen Hagan for the Canadian fun at CanFitPro; Carol for ECA; Bernard Hasse (for redefining 'LOVE' for me); Irene "Cathy" Narvaez (for the hundreds of e-mails as a premium personal assistant); Liz Kalmanowicz (for keeping the money flowing); Kathy Shelton for the first inspiration of excitement in my life (truly, my first friend), Lyndsay Murray-Kashoid for the great editing assistance, all of the colleagues who have come to any fitness session of mine at any convention anywhere; and Barbara.

ABCs INDEX...

A	Alignment & Abdominals	O	Observation
B	Breathing	P	Proprioception
C	Cardiovascular Fitness	Q	Quitting
D	Diets	R	Resistance & Strength training
E	Exercise & Endorphins	S	Spot reducing
F	Flexibility	T	Trilogy of fitness
G	Goals	U	Understanding the Information Out There
H	Hiring a trainer	V	Vitamins, minerals, & supplements
I	Intensity	W	Water
J	Joy	X	Xanadu
K	Keeping On Track	Y	Yoga
L	Logging, Lapses, & Laughter	Z	Zen
M	Machines		
N	New		

SPECIAL NOTE: FOR CONTINUOUSLY UPDATED
SUPPLEMENTAL INFORMATION ON THE ABC'S
OF FITNESS, PLEASE VISIT
WWW.FINDLAWRENCE.COM AND CLICK
'FREE STUFF'

INTRODUCTION

Welcome to my *ABCs of Fitness*! In grade school, I was an over fat, overfed, and under-exercised youth. I dedicated my time to both studying and eating. In 1983, after I graduated high school, my father died of heart disease. Years later, my mother needed open heart surgery to replace a defective valve, and in 2001, my only brother died instantly of a heart attack at work. I learned early in college that I, too, needed to heed the serious lessons that heredity held for me: a propensity to be round, to have high cholesterol, and to inherit heart disease.

Nobody's fitness suggestions made sense to me. Books seemed complicated. Sports seemed too intense. Nutritional advice seemed impossible to heed. Television told me to do something on one channel but on yet another someone wanted me to purchase a magic machine. Instead of making a choice to follow any one of those fitness pieces of advice, I chose instead to feel the "full and satisfied" feelings that came from eating a half-gallon of chocolate-chip mint ice cream after school while doing my homework. Years later after having found the right mentors with the right answers, I changed my body by deciding accept the truth: there is no magic pill, machine, or even book that will solve anything in fitness without my own hard commitment to be dedicated to change. To help others with my story, I decided to author a book using language that I could understand, putting together simple truths in an 'a, b, c' format.

Fortunately for me, I found a few mentors who could put positive lifestyle changes into little, simple steps for me. I thus decided to take strong control about my meals and my exercise regime and, before long, couldn't contain my enthusiasm. In the early 80's, I began sharing my exercises with individuals in personal training settings at a time when the non-profit and government-recognized American Council on Exercise (ACE) was preparing to launch its first internationally-accepted certifications. When ACE developed its first certification, I was in the first group ever to sit down and take it in Washington, DC. When I passed, I was 'gold certified,' meaning that I was among this first passing group of individuals. Of course, since those early days of industry-accepted certifications, other certifying bodies have also emerged. As a result, I got certified by them as well. (With pride I announce that, years later in 2002, the American Council on Exercise named me their Group Fitness Instructor of the Year!) I now serve on the Advisory Board to the American Council on Exercise and act as National Spokesperson for ACE's mission of helping people separate mindfulness from myth and fact from fiction in regards to fitness information

At university, I formed small groups with fellow students and even my professors, sharing with them how to exercise. Since those early days, I've enjoyed seeing fitness evolve. What we definitely agree on now is that *little* changes can reap *huge* benefits in one's life. Remember this: if you do nothing else in your life but take one flight of stairs instead of the moving escalator the next time you see the decision, you are making a step in the right direction towards moving towards wellness. Like one of my mentors from Reebok Annette Lang says, "Just move more!"

In the world of teaching group exercise classes and personal training, I've seen that so many instructors and trainers around the planet are popular, but it's important to make sure that they are currently certified as proof of their knowledge and ability. Instructors and trainers should be both popular and professional. It's easy to find some who are one or the other, but more of a challenge to find both.

Since I began teaching fitness in 1983, over the years people have asked me the same questions about fitness. We haven't changed in our fitness concerns. Questions such as "How do I loose the fat around my middle,?" "Can you just give me a diet to lose weight?" "What's the best exercise to lose fat,?", and "Can I really not eat any carbohydrates after 6pm? What is a carbohydrate anyway?" have plagued me for years. I think that, in the US alone, Americans have been on a diet for over twenty years and have done nothing successful but *gain fat.* Across the globe, despite years, ages, and even languages, the common concerns to us all remain unchanged. What follows is a list I've complied of these common questions from you since 1983. I've organized them according to the alphabet. Thank you for letting me share this information with you.

When you see TRY THIS: throughout this book, that's a time to understand before moving forward. In order to do this, it's best to FEEL the concept. Get ready to move during these sections, and know that skipping them will mean you will take less benefit from the book than if you make yourself try the simple tasks. Confucius said "I listen and I hear, I look and I see, but only when I *do* can I understand because I *feel.*" These are wise words. So promise yourself you will make time to TRY THIS every time you find that invitation from me in this book.

Whether you are deconditioned, new-to-fitness, or even a trained athlete, I hope that this book will shed some sane sense on the overall quality of your life. Nobody has to live in a gym to be fit and healthy. Remember the most exciting news of all is that even really little changes can reap big benefits in the body, so even choosing to park just a bit farther away from the mall than normal can lead you towards having a profound impact in your life far after you leave the mall! The take-home message of this book is this: *small changes can reap huge benefits, so the smallest change today definitely will increase the overall quality of your life tomorrow.*

This humble dictionary comes to you with a simple purpose which is my mission statement:

> *to help you orchestrate and coordinate movement and fitness into your life based on* **fact** *(and not on the common madness of misunderstandings so rampant in the media)*

Published information by the American Council on Exercise in their *Personal Training* and *Group Fitness Instructor* manuals tells us that nature-- these genetics we inherit from our parents-- partially determines our build throughout our lives. There are three main body types on the planet among all cultures, called somatotypes (sometimes called morphotypes): *ectomorphs* (delicately built individuals like Nicole

Kidman), *mesomorphs* (muscular and athletic like Arnold Schwarzenneger), and *endomorphs* (softer, rounder bodies with a propensity towards difficulty at losing weight like Oprah Winfrey). These three broad categories of body types were created in the early 1940s, not by a physician or exercise specialist, but by American psychologist William H. Sheldon. He reported on it in his book *The Varieties of Temperament,* which remains a classic book on body types for both the medical and the psychological professions. Sheldon, who died in 1977, developed his somatotypes theory after studying 4,000 photographs of college-age men. His primary research interest was drawing connections between body type and temperament. He theorized that ectomorphic people tend to be quiet and reflective; mesomorphs brim with energy and vigor; and endomorphic people are magnanimous and love to eat. While those connections play a relatively minor role in modern psychology and greatly oversimplify people, Sheldon's body types continue to influence how people exercise, body-build, and manage their weight. Years later, Carol Saltus published *Bodyscopes* in which she took these ideas a step further, discussing combinations of the original 3 somatotypes. She explains that, although genetics predetermine what general type you will have for life, proper training methods can produce desired changes within a framework of realistic goals. I want to emphasize that my purpose here is not to label you, for indeed, many of us are **combinations** of different body types. The important thing to remember is that you can't pick up a magazine and find the body type of someone you like and say "I'm going to work out until I have this guy's frame." Genetically inside of us is predetermined how our body will respond to fitness. Yes, we will definitely become healthier, but we cannot determine the shape of the bicep when we exercise it, for example. We can make it stronger, more functional, more lean, but we can't determine its ultimate shape. Just being aware of this genetic makeup fact will help you understand your predisposition to a particular body type, but this is only half of the story. What you choose to **do** with that makeup is all up to you.

Which body type would you fit into? *The Group Exercise Instructor Manual* of the American Council on Exercise states that everyone starts with these genetic predispositions. Exercise and meal plans can help make changes to small or moderate degrees. According to Joseph Cotton, editor for the aforementioned ACE industry standard textbook, no matter what you do, it is difficult, if not impossible, to change the body **type** you inherited from your parents. You can, however, move toward a **fitter level** within that particular type --if you are willing to put in the time. This means that, while you most definitely can add cardiovascular, strength, and flexibility training to your regime and improve the constitution of your body, you cannot "become" like another individual of a different body type. Jim Carey will never have the body of Arnold Schwarzenneger, for example.

Now that we've explored the two branches of us: what we are born with and what we can do with it, let's get started. Here's a toast to you and to a simple understanding of simple fitness truths. Weclome/Namaste!

A

ALIGNMENT & ABDOMINALS

Common Question: Why does my lower back always hurt?

Our energy starts with the way we align our spine, the long column of bones that resembles a series of doughnuts running up the back. Deviations that occur with muscular imbalances in certain parts of our back pull our spine too much in any one way, and we may experience this as pain, as a decrease in function when moving, or both. In India, yoga practitioners sometimes date themselves more on the age of their spine (and its healthy ability to move) than on chronological age, saying "you are as old as your spine is mobile." I like to rephrase that to "we are as *young* as our spine has mobility." Alignment" means that when standing, the major joints (as well as a few special landmarks like ears) all follow an imaginary, minimally-curved line connecting ear to shoulder to mid-chest to hip to knee to ankle.

Look at yourself sideways in a mirror, and see if these landmarks line up. (*You really have to put this book down now and try it: you cannot learn anything about yourself if you just read these sentences!*) It may be best to have someone read the following aloud to you as you watch yourself from the side. "Try to adjust your body so the center of your ear lines up directly over the center of your shoulder, and they in turn line up over the hips, over the knees, and over the ankles. Imagine a line that connects the ears, shoulders, hips, knees, and ankles. The chin should point towards the floor. Take a step forward and a step backward while maintaining this position. Although it may not feel comfortable, this is the most aligned position for all of your joints, muscles, and bones."

This standing alignment is also referred to as neutral, or "anatomical position." Try to sit down in a straight-backed chair and maintain this same alignment, with only the knees coming out of that imaginary line. This means that your ears are still over your shoulders, which line up over the bony parts of the hips. Then there should be another imaginary vertical line connecting the knees to the ankles. When you sit, notice how these landmarks still follow alignment, but now you have angles as the knees and hips have bent. There are still long lines that connect the landmarks we just discussed. In 'neutral,' nothing is twisted or rotated. Healthy individuals learn how to train the parts of their bodies always starting and finishing in neutral. The point is that, regardless of what you do in life, from bending to gardening to sleeping, being aware of these lines and curves that connect the body is the starting place to keep you healthy.

To be sure, during daily life activities, you will move in and out of neutral, but always coming back to neutral can help your spine 'regain' its alignment. When aligned, the spine is at its strongest. Imbalances come when we make movements that move the body out of alignment, such as raising one shoulder higher than another when carrying a bag of groceries on one side of the body, for example.

TRY THIS:

Try these drills now: Stand in the alignment you found before and throw a book or towel on the floor without bending down. Now the task is to get it, to pick it up, without curving the spine *because curving the spine towards the floor from a standing position definitely puts great amounts of stress on the spine.* Think about squatting down, bending your knees and hips as if you were going to sit on the toilet or a chair, keeping your head and chest high. Keep bending your knees until you can reach forward with your arms to pick up the object, *without* bending the spine. It may take practice, and it may take doing this in front of a mirror.

Finally, practice "sucking in," pulling your belly button in the direction of the spine as if someone were going to take a picture of you in a bathing suit...you want to be thin in the picture, so you squeeze. One of the most important techniques to support the spine is this 'drawing in' maneuver.

TRY THIS:

Put one hand over your belly button area and spread your fingers to cover as much of your front core as possible. With the other hand, squeeze both nostrils and try to blow out your air. You will feel the lower part of your core contract inwards. This is another example of how to feel the 'drawing in' maneuver so important in protecting the core. Now, repeat the exercises in the previous paragraphs for the spine with this 'drawing in' action and notice how much stronger you feel as you use your abdominals to support your alignment! *This very act of "compression" is the single most important thing you can do to protect the spine when exerting force. Why not make it your new habit?*

This spine, by the way is not straight; it has curves that we should celebrate as we grow. Being told to "sit up straight" as children most likely came with the best intentions of our parents or guardians. However, know that sitting up "tall," "long," "lengthened," "proud," or "extended" are much more specific cues. The goal is to use all of the muscles in your body to "turn on" and activate a better posture as you try to grow taller. Using all of your muscles along your spine to maintain this spinal alignment requires work! Think about it: if you totally relaxed and turned your muscles off as you read this book, wouldn't you slump into a little ball on the floor? That means that obviously some muscles are alive and at work just so you can maintain a position to read this book.

Since life consists of a variety of movements that require the spine to move in different ways, we should celebrate all of the movements that the spine can make: bending forward (forward flexion), bending backwards (extension), bending sideways (lateral flexion), and twisting (rotation). If we spend a little time training these movements, we can help ourselves be champions of living and avoid injury during these movements in activities of daily life. Try to find at least one exercise for each of those movements and practice it each day to keep the spine moving freely.

To get you started, sit "tall" in a chair noticing the alignment we just discussed. Keep breathing comfortably during each of the following exercises.

FLEXION (means "bending forward"):

Next, walk your hands down your legs to touch your ankles, feet, or toes. Feel your back stretch. This is an example of flexion. Slowly return to sitting.

EXTENSION (means "bending backwards"):

Next, place your palms on your lower back (or the back of the chair) and try to bend a bit backwards, raising your chest towards the sky without dropping the head backwards as if you were watching a plane fly overhead. Feel the stretch down the front of the body. This is an example of extension.

LATERAL FLEXION (means "bending to the side"):

Next, raise one arm into the air while the other reaches towards the floor until you feel a stretch down one side and bend sideways just a bit. Repeat to the other side. This is an example of lateral flexion.

ROTATION (means "twisting"):

Finally, sit up tall and extend your elbows, reaching your hands towards the sides of the room. Slowly rotate (twist) in one direction, avoiding the temptation to slouch as you rotate. Feel some muscles pulling you into rotation and some muscles stretching. Repeat to the other side. This is an example of rotation.

You'll be surprised how young you remain as you maintain the suppleness and health of your spine. In each of these aforementioned examples of spinal exercises, you are working your abdominal muscles in slightly different ways, to boot!

These abdominal muscles are our center of power and work to support our marvelous spine. Having great 'abdominals' means being able to work both the abdominals (many separate muscles) and muscles that assist them, the back muscles as well! It means you can do all the "functions" of daily life using them to protect the spine in all of the movements we just discussed. This is what we mean by 'functional training' in the fitness industry. We help people understand how the spine works so that every movement of daily life, from filling the clothes drier to putting an airplane carry-on in an overhead bin, becomes easier and safer.

The function of your abdominals is more important than what people can see when you wear a bathing suit, for example. Just having "six-pack" lines in the abdominal area does not guarantee that one has functional abdominals: they have to be able to both tolerate and generate force for daily activities. Furthermore, we have already seen that genetics have predetermined how much of a 'six-pack' you will show with training. The good news, however, is that you can control the speed, efficiency, and execution of specific exercises, as well as modify the percentage of body fat around those muscles by adjusting how and what you consume.

Most people think that "working" their abdominals requires doing hundreds of crunches and then hundreds more. I'd rather you work smarter, not harder, and work from the inside out. No published research documents the need for excessive crunching actions for the spine. Please aim for quality instead of quantity on your abdominal exercises.

TRY THIS:

Lay supine (face up) on the floor and find neutral alignment so that your ribs and hips feel like there is space between them without the ribs "boinking" or popping up. This means that they are connected by an imaginary girdle of strength. This is still the connection you have when standing with the imaginary line among ears, shoulders, hips, knees, and ankles. The lower back should remain relaxed with a small, natural curve. Bend your knees so that your feet are as wide as your hips at a comfortable distance from your glutes. At no time during the exercise should we increase or decrease the space between the lower back and the floor, and this often happens when the spine arches backwards as people begin to crunch. Let's avoid that. Have someone read the following as you try.

"To begin, squeeze the muscles that control body elimination of solids and liquids. This is different from 'drawing in' maneuver that pulls in the circumference of the waist. This closes and controls the pelvic floor area, a necessary function to promote stability in men and women. It's the most center part of your core that you can control. Maintain that activation of these deep pelvic core muscles because this will keep your spine healthier, your posture improved, and your center ("core") stable. This is the true heart of 'core training.' Second, activate the next muscles we want to target called the 'transverse abdominus' by drawing the navel in, up, and wide towards the spinal column. Imagine that you have a lemon and you put that between your belly button and spine. Compress downwards and make lemonade! Concentrating on your breath, prepare to exhale and tuck your chin gently towards your chest as you allow the lowest ribs--ever so slowly-- to approach the hip bones as you raise your upper body from the floor. The shoulder blades may just lift off of the floor slightly. Lower back to where you began with the same speed and control. Make sure that you exhale on the phase when you move upwards away from the floor. The head keeps its relationship with the neck at all times, so the chin never should get closer to the chest at any specific time. Try a few contractions on a diagonal in which the right shoulder travels in the direction of the left knee, and vice-versa. Try each movement as slow as possible, starting with at least 5 repetitions of each. The hands can lay by the hips, cross the chest, or support the head as long as the arms do not pull on the head. The elbows should remain behind the head, out of peripheral vision, at all times."

TRY THIS:

Again, have someone read to you the following: "In order to work the opposing muscles of the back, the spinal erectors that run from the neck to the hips, lay face down with the hands at the hips. Face the floor at all times, never looking forwards or up. As you exhale, lift the head, neck, and as much of the chest as you can off of the floor, and slowly lower. Think of doing the same movement as in the previous exercise, only behind you: take the lowest ribs towards the back hip bones. At no time should the feet leave the floor, and the eyes always maintain focused on the floor, never forwards, to ensure the neck remains in alignment. To be sure you are doing this correctly, put a tennis ball or small round fruit between your chin and chest. Keep it there for the remainder of the exercise; if it falls towards the floor, you know you have lost the important alignment of the neck. Try each movement as slow as possible to start for at least 5 repetitions of each."

Many of the common aches and pains in the lower back can be alleviated by developing balance and strength of both the abdominal and back muscles. When one is over or underdeveloped, alignment is skewed and certain muscles remain in a constant state of tension, while others lengthen reducing the overall structural stability. This puts joints in a compromised position making injury more likely. This postural imbalance also accounts for the additional pull and tightness in the area of the lower spine. Keeping the abdominals and back strong will make sure you always come into and out of alignment in the safest way possible, ensuring a healthy, functional life!

Being aware that your spine truly is your backbone in life will help you train it. Remember that you have 7 bones of the back in your neck, called cervical vertebrae. In the middle of the back, you have 12, called the thoracic vertebrae. Around your belt line, you have 5 more called the lumbar vertebrae. Finally, you have a tailbone. You can remember how many vertebrae you have from top to bottom if you remember the mealtimes of most Americans: breakfast at 7, lunch at 12, and dinner at 5! Truly, you will be as healthy as your spine. I conclude with an invitation back to you: "Tell me how healthy is your spine and I will tell you how healthy is your life."

B

BREATHING

Common Questions: Why am I always out of breath? Why don't I sleep well? Why should I even think about my breathing?

When your breathing muscles around and below the ribs are fit and strong, you are able to process more oxygen with each breath. When this happens, you are able to do more of life's daily tasks more efficiently without finding yourself out of breath. This breathing efficiency is called "VO2 max" in scientific terms, 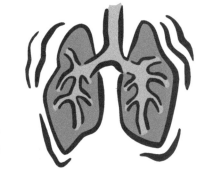 and it means that the higher your VO2 max number, the stronger you are in the upper chest and back part of your core for using oxygen for daily activities.

Breathing exercises are commonly used for treatment of insomnia, panic disorders, migraines, chronic pains, etc. A balanced nervous system promotes overall well-being, including favorable sleeping patterns.

According to ancient texts our breath is our source of life. An ancient Hindu saying states "He or she who half breathes, only half lives." This shows us the importance of getting the most out of our lives by getting the most out of the quality of each breath. (In Hindi: "Jho insaan thota sash leja thoda jeeyaygaa; jho inshaan poora sash lega poora jeeyagaa").

Granted, breathing for most of us isn't something we think about on a daily basis, but stopping occasionally to think about the quality of the breaths we take can increase the quality of our lives. If you can think about your breath, you can increase its quality of inhalation and exhalation (length and depth). If you increase the quality you can nourish the body with more oxygen. If you nourish the body with more oxygen, you assist and facilitate the many functions dependent on oxygen like elimination of toxins, manufacture of ATP (energy in the body used for all work), and daily function of internal organs. Everything we do begins and ends with breathing. It's the first thing we've done on the planet, and it will be the last thing we do, no matter how we leave.

There are about ten different breathing techniques, with even more variations within each of them. One of the most essential requires an understanding that the nose is on the face for the purpose of breathing, and the mouth is more naturally designed for communication and feeding. The nose is responsible for purifying and warming air before it reaches the lungs. Notice how babies and dogs breathe through their noses when they sleep, which shows us this natural state. Over time as we age, we sometimes lose that ability to process our breathing via our noses due to accidents, surgeries, changes in health and immune system strength, among other things.

TRY THIS:

To deepen a sense of awareness and relaxation of the breath, sit tall and place one hand over the chest and another on the belly area, over the belly button. Try to inhale deep and long through the nose, feeling the air fill under both hands. Perhaps you can count up to three as you inhale, counting up: "one, two, three." Exhale now, and let the air leave your body via the nose, counting in reverse, "three, two, one." Try to feel movement under both hands as the air leaves under them. Think of the action of filling a tall glass pitcher with lemonade, where your lungs are the pitcher. As you inhale, fill the bottom of the pitcher first (your diaphragm, deep belly area, and low chest), and then follow the movement up the torso as you fill your "pitcher" with air. Feel your lower hand expand and move first, filling with air, and then your top hand. When you exhale through the nose, think of pouring out the "lemonade," or air in the natural way it would leave the pitcher: from the top first, the from the middle, and then from the lower parts of the pitcher/lungs, just in reverse order from your filling process. When you exhale, then, you feel the air leave under the top hand first, then from the lower hand.

Another technique for nose breathing helps you direct air to the back of your lungs, an often unused section.

TRY THIS:

Lay face up on the floor or a bed. Bend your knees to feel comfortable in the lower back area, with the feet as wide as the hips, on the floor or bed. Place your hands around your ribcage with your thumbs wrapped under you towards the floor, over your back ribs. As you inhale through the nose, feel your fingers expand as the muscles between your ribs, and the ribs themselves, expand with air. Try to feel that expansion against your thumbs in back of you as your back ribs expand. After a few minutes, turn over face down, and turn your head to one side to keep a neutral neck. Place your hands by your sides with your thumbs facing the floor, under you, and your fingers wrapped around your ribcage, towards the ceiling. With the exception of your thumbs, your fingers are on your low to mid- back. Relax any tension in your shoulders. As you inhale in this position, concentrate on feeling your back ribs expand now, more than you felt before when you were supine, or face up. Because the floor or bed is under you, it's more difficult for the lungs to expand to the front and easier for them to expand towards the rear. Feel your body rise and fall as you breathe through the nose, and imagine that you are getting more oxygen to the back parts of the lungs.

After a few minutes, you may feel a renewed sense of awareness about your body because you've made breathing, if only for a moment, a conscious act. Furthermore, you have awakened your sense of awareness about the ribs and lungs, and you have become more aware of directing air to the back of the body when breathing. Getting more air to the mind and muscles always is a good thing because this helps them function more efficiently, and usually we can also think, relax, digest, and even sleep better!

C

CARDIOVASCULAR FITNESS

STRENGTH   FLEXIBILITY

Common Question: What's the best
exercise for me to lose weight?

Cardiovascular fitness is one of the
three angles of our fitness trilogy triangle:
cardiovascular, strength, and flexibility. It
refers to the blood and oxygen both
 coming to, and leaving
from, the heart muscle
(the "cardio" of the title)
and the lungs. The
"vascular" refers to the
arteries and veins
through which the
blood flows to get
from the heart to the
muscles and back.
Because blood gets 'tired"
and needs 'refreshing' like filters that
purify room air, the blood travels through
the lungs for this exchange and 'service

station.' The harder you work and start puffing air, the more you work the heart and lungs for this exchange to occur, and the more you nourish the brain and body with good oxygen. Other benefits include the heart getting stronger and more efficient as a pump, so it has to beat less per minute as it pushes more blood and oxygen throughout your body. This means that, over time, a person who becomes fit will have a *lower* heart rate than before because the heart becomes extremely efficient.

TRY THIS:

Take your heart rate now for one full minute if you've been resting and reading this. If you have not been resting, sit for 20 minutes and then take your pulse by using your fingers just to the side of your Adam's apple (not your thumb, though, because it has its own pulse which you'll feel) until you feel the pulse alongside of your neck. To find your pulse easily, look up gently to stretch the skin in your neck and feel around for the pulse. Count it for 60 seconds and record it in the following chart.

Take this again every two weeks and see if you notice any difference. Normal pulses vary between 70-80 beats per minute in non-exercisers, but people with healthy, efficient hearts can have really low pulse rates! If you make small changes to your lifestyle including exercise, you may notice that your resting heart pulse comes down, which is a great sign that your heart is becoming more efficient at pumping *more* blood with each contraction and having to beat *less*.

Date	Pulse Beats in 60 Seconds

What's the best cardiovascular exercise? All respected researchers agree that the best is the one you are willing to do for the most amount of time, with the most amount of regularity, with the most enjoyment! The 50 calories from walking or stepping or dancing or swimming or gardening are the same calories used and burned, but the muscles used may be different. If your purpose is to lose fat (also see "Spot Reducing"), then find cardiovascular exercises that work for you!

We have to make the heart work harder, called cardiovascular training, because it uses fat as a fuel during its work. We want to burn fat, so cardiovascular training proves worthy. Aerobic exercises –this intense work that makes us breathe heavily-- increases the amount of oxygen available to the body, and on a cellular level this translates to an increase in fat burning metabolism! Be patient. Sometimes it seems like where we want to lose the fat we've gained, it comes off last. At the very least, try walking at a moderate pace for ten minutes for your cardiovascular exercise. If knee health is an issue, try cycling in one of the recumbent (reclining) bicycles that are so popular in most gyms.

Every few weeks, think about changing the type of cardiovascular exercise you've chosen, just to 'wake up' your muscles and teach them to react in new ways. This means creating new neuromuscular pathways which keeps your muscles on their toes! You can always return to your favorite cardiovascular exercise after you try varying something once or twice. The body does need change periodically, but just be sure that your cardiovascular choices are safe for you.

D

DIETS

Common Question: Can you just give me a
diet so I can lose weight?

Everywhere I go, as soon as people
learn I am in fitness, people ask me: "Can
you just give me a diet?" Diets connote
short-term periods of time. Diets are also
something Americans tend to go "onto"
and "fall off of" often. They are temporary,
short-lived, wreaked with fads, and often
unimpressive. Since we eat for life as a
long term plan, and since diets connote
short-term plans, it seems reasonable that
we should rethink the concept of 'diet'
completely. Instead of 'diet," I prefer the
term 'meal plan' because it's a concept
that doesn't intimidate us when we think
of following it for life. Meal plans take into
consideration each individual's realistic
goals, tastes, likes and dislikes, and
applicability to daily life.
One size does not fit all.
For example, suggesting
a meal plan that
consists of breakfasts of
quinoa-based waffles,
lowfat yogurt with sliced

and peeled fruit, and a flaxseed power smoothie may be nutritionally sound for one gentleman who offices out of home because he has a kitchen nearby, but suggesting that same breakfast meal plan to a woman who travels frequently on planes during the breakfast hour would be a recipe for failure. Cultural differences, medical needs, and lifestyle choices often affect meal plans.

Individuals with specific medical reasons for consulting a specialist should consult Registered Dieticians. If you are serious about finding one in your area, consult www.eatright.org, the website of the nonprofit American Dietetic Association. Even though you may see the word 'Diet" as part of the title, rest assured that the website has to do with all aspects of sound, researched nutrition that helps increase the quality of peoples' lives everyday. It is not a website about 'dieting!' A Registered Dietician can help you create innovate, realistic, and do-able meal plans that can work for you to help you achieve the realistic goals you want.

As the ACE *Personal Training* and *Group Fitness Manuals* state, the body needs about 55% of carbohydrates, 15% of proteins, and up to 30% of fat at every meal or snack. An example of this from the Mediterranean style of eating could be white or whole wheat pasta (healthy carbohydrate choices with some protein) topped with tomato sauce with olive oil (healthy choices of fat), mixed with strips of lean chicken, beef, pork, or fish (lean protein choices).

When people ask me what I eat on any given day, I'm happy to tell them. After I explain what I've ingested, I always follow that up with a breakdown of how active I am, what my general medical needs are, and why I choose the foods I do based on my travel schedule for that given week. It's important for people to realize that they shouldn't follow my meal plans because we are different people with different physical needs, cultural backgrounds, lifestyles, and travel schedules. When it comes to supplementation ("Should I take vitamins?"), the American Council on Exercise suggests that we always refer clients to their medical care practitioners for supplementation recommendations because only the doctors know things like the results of blood work, possible vitamin-medicine interactions, family history, etc.

Fat often gets a bad reputation. Fat provides great functions in the body: it carries some vitamins like A, D, E, and K, stimulates growth, protects organs, regulates heat, and helps the body digest every type of food. Carrying too much fat on the body, especially when that fat accumulates around the center of the individual, puts an increase risk for cardiovascular disease on that individual. Eliminating total fat intake is not the way to decrease fat storage on the body, however, because we need some fat everyday just to survive. Just the gallbladder alones needs roughly ten grams of fat at every full meal just to engage in all of its functions properly. Getting healthy fat from sound sources in the right amounts is key.

Read labels. Look for ingredients that say "monounsaturated" and "polyunsaturated" types of fats. You want these.

Limit "saturated" fats (fats, like lard, that come from animals) as much as possible. Learn the words "hydrogenated," "partially hydrogenated," "trans fat," "fractionated" and try to eliminate from your grocery purchases all foods listing these words in the ingredients, because this process of hydrogenation can increase your risk for cardiac and other diseases. You do not want these.

I'd like to share two final thoughts regarding food meal plans. First, there are no real 'junk foods,' because the body can tolerate almost anything in the appropriate quantity. While there are no junk foods, from listening to what people have been telling me for so many years, I do believe that there are some really junky meal plans. Potato chips in small amounts won't ruin anybody, for example, but if that's *all* you eating over time, then your meal plan is really junky. Although it's also a trite slogan, it really proves true!

Remember not to equate ethics and morality with food. We don't behave 'good' or 'bad' when we eat certain things. We are 'good' and 'bad' based on our actions in society. We may follow a healthy meal plan or not, but it doesn't change who we are inside in terms of morality. From my good friend and Hollywood Registered Dietician Dominique Adair, I suggest using the word 'bad' in relation to food only when a food has spoiled or we are allergic to it. Spoiled milk truly has gone "bad." This keeps morality out of food, and will keep us from thinking negative thoughts based on what we have or have not ingested. If we eat an apple or piece of chocolate, therefore, neither makes us 'good' nor 'bad.'

E

 EXERCISE & ENDORPHINS

Common question: "I don't do anything....so how do I start?"

Exercise sounds like a generic term that could describe just about anything involving movement, and the truth is that it almost can! The best exercise is whatever you are willing to do with the best form and most dedication! Remember, though, that there is a trilogy of fitness (see "C" and "T") as you choose, so we have to choose exercises that address, to some degree, flexibility training, cardiovascular training, and strength training. One general rule for exercise:

> *training you do for either flexibility, cardiovascular, or strength for at least ten minutes at a time with proper form and execution to increase (or maintain) your fitness level.*

Exercise can improve the overall quality of your life in many ways, including making your heart, lungs, muscles, and even organs stronger and more efficient. Exercise helps rid your body of toxins, helps you sleep better, and can act like nature's caffeine by boosting your own natural energy levels that start in the brain, called endorphins. These *endorphins* are chemicals released in the brain that make you happier by elevating mood naturally and make you want more. In the beginning phases of exercise, however, the muscles first get sore, so be sure to read "Q"! Finally, please remember that exercise does not mean that you must replicate what you see on television or at your local gym. Exercise can be as aggressive as 'boot camp' callisthenic classes or as simple as pruning the shrubs in your back yard.

The U.S. Surgeon General has made a statement that it's best for us to get at least one hour of movement activity on all or most days of the week. This can be challenging for the person who by nature is inactive, so I urge you to think in small terms. In the beginning, just try to do some movement-based activity for 10 minutes. This will automatically increase as you reap the benefits of fitness and start to notice differences. So get out and garden, pick up weeds, clean out an old closet with high and low shelves, take a short walk, or do anything that involves movement: it can involve strength, cardiovascular exercise, or flexibility. Remember, the key word is *"movement."*

F

FLEXIBILITY

Common question: "I'm not into yoga.
How do I stretch, and why?"

Flexibility keeps muscles healthy, and refers to a muscle's ability to get longer when it needs to be able to change length. The purpose of working on flexibility is to prevent injury, help your posture, and balance those other parts of our fitness trilogy (strength and cardiovascular exercise) which tend to make muscles tighter and shorter. Flexibility can increase the overall quality of your life by making sure that muscles and bones can react to different movements (tensions) during the activities of daily life. When movement around joints, called "flexibility," is ample, then there is decreased risk for injury because the body moves with more efficiency. When connections are tight, the risk for injury rises and simple movements like picking up fallen car keys could overstretch the back, putting you out of commission for many days because your muscles aren't flexible enough to support the change in posture against gravity when you bend down and then return. Flexibility does not always feel good; the tighter we are, the worse it can feel when we stretch. A safe guideline for stretching, therefore, is to find a point of discomfort that is not pain and hold that position of stretch for at least 20 seconds. If you can repeat this several times in a single stretching session, the American Council on Exercise tell us we are likely to see more results than just stretching periodically.

The best way to stretch is to learn how to put the body in a position that keeps it neutral and supported so the muscles you are trying to stretch can elongate while the rest of your body remains in the alignment we discuss in "A." Notice in the photo how the upper body is supported while the emphasis is on stretching the muscles in the back of the lower leg behind the body. T'ai Chi, yoga 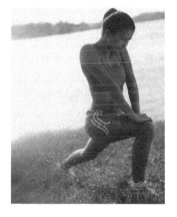 and Pilates (pronounced /pi-lah-tease/) are mindful forms of exercise that really help your muscular flexibility. Sometimes you may see runners outside stretching before and after their activity. If you see a runner holding a stretch (with no observable movement) rest assured this runner probably stretches appropriately. If, however, you see someone stretching and bouncing during a stretch, the potential for injury increases because this actually makes the muscles *shorter* instead of longer! Stretches should be slow and controlled with not much movement.

You can stretch muscles standing, sitting, and lying down, as long as you know what you're doing. Muscles stretch better when they are warm, so the best times to stretch are when your body is warm from a Jacuzzi, shower, bath, humid environment, or light movement exercise, for example. Waking up on a cold winter morning is not the best time to stretch without doing a bit of movement first to warm up those muscles, even if that means walking around for a minute.

Stretches that incorporate the whole body can be done on the floor. It's a great place to start because the floor helps support and protect the body so there's less chance to fall, lose balance, or come out of alignment.

TRY THIS:

Lay on the floor or bed, face down, and come up onto the elbows, pushing the shoulders towards the floor and opening the knees as wide as the hips. Bend the knees so the feet come towards the sky. This stretches the muscles all along the front of the body: thighs (quadriceps), hips (hip flexors), and torso (abdominals and pectoralis major in the chest). For a balancing stretch for the muscles down the back of the body, come onto hands and knees from that position. Round the back so you look at your belly button, like an angry cat, lowering the head towards the pelvis without bending the elbows.

Flexibility in the body will increase your ability to do daily functions and help prevent injury. Remember, though, that there are other types of flexibility that are important for your overall health. Flexibility of the mind can help you manage stress and you become able to bend your will and accept both things you cannot control and also the wishes of other people. Flexibility of our approach to different people, cultures, and ways of doing things can decrease stress as we cease trying to impose our will on the world. Flexibility of tolerance means that we allow for different styles of doing things that may not be congruent with our own, without judgment.

How will you develop your own flexibility?

G

GOALS

Common question: "I tried exercise. Why didn't I see any results to my goals?"

This section is short but powerful with only two take-home messages. These are secrets most people never discover.

First, those who write down their fitness goals are much more likely to achieve them. Be specific. Instead of writing "get healthier," break that down into smaller, measurable steps. For example: "lose one pound of fat in 2 weeks," "lose an inch of fat around my midsection," and "walk for 10 minutes per day to start for 5 days every week" are definite, measurable goals. Write them on sticky notes and display them prominently on your refrigerator, in your purse/wallet, car, and anywhere else you normally would have visual access. If you have access to a photocopy machine, make copies and post these goals everywhere. Remember, if you aren't committed enough to write down your goal, you most probably aren't committed enough to take the appropriate steps to achieve the goals themselves.

Second, fitness goals need to be *realistic* goals. The American Dietetic Association recommends that a healthy weight-loss plan, at best, can promote a loss of two pounds of fat per week. Be wary of any goals that promise above that.

I always joke as mind-body personal trainer when individuals come to me with a picture of a Hollywood model in one hand and a size 2 dress or suit in the other and tell me that these are their fitness goals. We've seen that one of the determining factors in achieving our realistic goals is our inherited, genetic makeup: what our ancestors have bestowed upon us. Each body type can make marvelous changes in increasing the quality of life through flexibility, cardiovascular, and strength training, but only to certain maximum degrees. For example, in my case I know that I'll never be Hercules in muscular size, no matter how I try, so I train well the body type I have and learn to love what I train!

In achieving fitness goals, the most important thing is to know the purpose of any flexibility, cardiovascular, and strength exercise. If you don't know the purpose, please don't do it until you do, and be sure that the purpose makes sense and gets you closer to your goal.

Re-evaluate your fitness goals often, and share this with experts in fitness. Also, if you write them down, you are more likely to achieve them!

Use this space below to think about goals.

Something I wanted to do in my past that I set out to do and achieve was:

What helped me do that was:

Something that I want to do in my future is:

Things that can help me achieve that are:

H

HIRING A FITNESS CONSULTANT/PERSONAL TRAINER

Common Question: "How do I know if a personal trainer is right for me, and how do I find one?"

Personal Trainers can help motivate and educate! It costs nothing to begin a search of personal trainers in your area that would make you feel comfortable. Before you search, some honest self-searching can prove useful. Begin by trying to fill out the following chart as honestly as you can.

About me:

MY realistic goals by 2 weeks:	
MY realistic goals by 4 weeks:	
MY realistic goals by 6 months:	
MY realistic goals by 1 year:	
Changes I want to feel in my body:	
Changes I want to see in my body:	
Habit changes I want to make: (eating, sleeping, working, working out, ...)	
Find out more about: (food, exercises, weights, things I've seen on tv,..)	

As you search for a currently-certified personal trainer, the website of the American Council on Exercise (www.acefitness.org) can help you locate a certified personal trainer in your area of the world. Their logo looks like this:

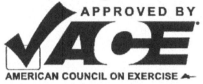

Other sites to help you search include www.afaa.com, www.nasm.org, www.acsm.com, and www.equinoxfitness.com.

When you begin calling fitness facilities in your area looking for specific, nationally-certified trainers, ask for the best personal trainer based on the goals you listed above. If you are just beginning in fitness, your personal trainer will be able to help you define these better because sometimes we don't know exactly what's realistic to expect at the start. Oftentimes, it takes a professional to be able to ascertain what's feasible. Ask for a suggestion of the person best suited for you based on that, and be sure to show your answers above with him or her.

Professional and ethical personal trainers and group fitness instructors not only get certified by internationally-recognized sources, but they *maintain* their certifications with a minimum of fifteen hours of continuing education every two years. This is the importance of using your first meetings as a sort of job interview and of asking if your trainer is *currently* certified, not just certified. Current certification bears importance because research in fitness brings new information, and every client has the right to hire a personal trainer with the most updated information in his or her techniques and trends. You want a trainer using up-to-date methods based on research so that you get the maximum benefits in the minimum amount of your precious commodity of time.

Current USA standards for personal training certification recognize the American Council on Exercise (ACE), Aerobics and Fitness Association of America (AFAA), American College of Sports Medicine (ACSM), Cooper Institute for Aerobics Research (CIAR), National Academy of Sports Medicine (NASM), National Sports Conditioning Association (NSCA), and, exclusively for the aquatic environment, the Aquatic Exercise Association (AEA). International certification companies exist outside of the USA with excellent records. Always consult their websites to see what their trainers have to demonstrate in terms of proficiency before acquiring their certification.

Certifications for group fitness instructors (formerly referred to as "aerobics instructors") exist within these same organizations. You should protect yourself well by searching for classes taught by those group fitness instructors in your clubs who maintain current certifications from these organizations as well!

When making a decision to hire a personal trainer, try to give yourself at least two sessions before deciding that 'this person is or is not for me.' Make sure your certified trainer understands your goals and has explained how realistic they are. Furthermore, an excellent personal trainer changes your routine every few times you meet. You do not need to pay someone to coach you through exercise you know by heart and can do just as well on your own! If that were the case, you could just pop in your own DVD at home! The best personal trainers train to some degree your mind, body, and breath in every session. Remember, too, that you always can move on to another personal trainer or group fitness instructor if the fit just doesn't feel right.

Complacency can become negative for muscles. World-class, effective personal trainers always achieve two things: they help their clients feel successful at achieving their realistic goals, and they constantly change up exercise design so the clients' muscles never get bored or adapted to any particular set of stimuli. Research by Dr. Len Kravitz, Coordinator of Exercise

Science at the University of New Mexico, shows that muscles need constant change or else they adapt and change little (Overturf, R. & Kravitz, L. (2002). Strength training and flexibility. IDEA Personal Trainer, 13(8), 17-19.).

When you find your certified personal trainer with whom you actually begin working, establish an interview and make a note of the answers to the following questions. You should not feel like you are prying when inquiring because this is someone into whose hands you will place your livelihood. You will most likely spend many more hours than you ever would be spending with even your own medical health care practitioner! Search, interview, compare, and then decide.

Use the following chart on the next page as you interview prospective (or even current) personal trainers.

Finally, remember that a personal trainer can help you motivate, guide your exercise selection, and ensure safety. That said, it's important you know that success depends on you as no personal trainer is a magician! Promise to be honest with your trainer no matter what the story you tell: whether you lived in a fast food restaurant for 3 days or didn't do any assigned exercises: honesty will allow future work to be more profitable!

Personal Trainer Overview/Interview:

Name:	
Are you currently certified? By whom?	ACE AFAA ACSM CIAR NASM NSCA AEA Other?
How long have you been doing this?	
How much do you charge? (rate scale, 30 minute or 60 minute sessions, does pre-paying for some sessions give you an additional session free?)	
What is your cancellation policy? (including: how can I cancel if the fit just doesn't feel right?)	
Do you train in the gym or come to my home?	
What's the average age of your clients?	
Are your sessions 60 minutes or do you offer 30 minute sessions?	

I

INTENSITY

Common question: "How do I know how hard to train?"

This short section contains a powerful message: intensity tells us how hard we are working with relation to effort. To get faster results, increasing intensity is one factor you can manipulate. It is not necessary, however! Having a general idea of our intensity helps us meet our goals because we learn if we should increase or decrease our work effort. It also keeps us empowered by reminding us we are in constant control.

The Rating of Perceived Exertion is a wonderful tool for determining intensity because it helps train your mind and body by creating a brain-body connection. It consists of a scale between 6 and 20. Think of how you feel when you wake up on the morning where you can stay in bed without rush. This is a level 6 for almost everyone. Think of working so hard running up a steep mountain that you cannot continue anymore because you're completely exhausted. This is a level 20 for almost everyone. During our day, then, when we do different things, we should try to determine what numbers apply to our intensity and exertion. At different times of our days, sometimes we're at a 7, a 10, and 16, for example.

In the following chart, try to pick the number that best relates to where you are right now. Remember that at no number should you feel pain. These numbers help you understand how hard you are working. The colors also help you determine your intensity. 6-10 area means it's easy to do everything, and "go" like for a green traffic stoplight. The 11-16 range means you are working harder and should be mindful of the change in your intensity. 17-20 range means your intensity is high, which may or may not be your desired effect.

SCALE OF PERCEIVED EXERTION

6	Staying awake in bed
7	Sitting up in bed, talking, reading, eating
8	Walking to the kitchen, preparing breakfast
9	Cleaning up breakfast, loading the dishwasher, sweeping the kitchen floor
10	Taking a shower, starting to rake leaves, starting to perspire, feeling warmer
11	Working moderately hard, you take off a sweatshirt
12	Working moderately harder in a sustained manner; you can converse
13	Working moderately harder; more difficult to speak
14	Working hard; breathing usually is through the mouth exclusively
15	Working harder, sweat may be consistent
16	Working harder and feeling like it's 'hard'
17	Almost panting for breath, maybe sweating heavily
18	Working very hard
19	Working extremely hard, difficult to speak, maybe sweating profusely
20	Exhausted at the top of the hill

Can you determine your exercise intensity number at this moment? Try to use numbers, colors, and words to help you.

The purpose of finding a number of perceived intensity exertion is that, when you add a zero to that number, you know fairly accurately what your heart rate is as long as you are not on any medication that alters your heart rate. If you are, consult with your medical health care practitioner to learn how to make adjustments for your particular heart rate and find alternative ways to measure you pulse rate and interpret those numbers.

In the beginning, stay in the 6-10 area regardless what form of exercise you are choosing: strength, cardiovascular, or flexibility. You should move into 11-16 range as you get more fit, and into the 17-20 range after that. Easy does it! When you want to strength train and you are new to fitness, you will commence in the 6-10 area and progress towards the 11-16 range. The 17-20 zone is for people who have already achieved a high level of physical fitness and who need to push themselves to get even fitter in this way.

TRY THIS (with a calculator):

Fill in the blanks:

220 – (your age) = _____ (Example: if you are 20 years old, then you write "200" on the blank.

Multiply the number you put in the line above ____ by .60 = _____. We'll call this number (A)

Multiply the same number you put in the line above also by .90= _____ (B). We'll call this number (B).

You have two numbers now, (A) and (B). This is the range you want your heart to beat within when you practice cardiovascular exercise.

How do you know where your heart is beating? You can stop exercising and count the pulse, but this can be dangerous because your heart rate plummets when you stop abruptly. The easier way is to just use the chart above for an approximation, finding your number and adding a zero. The great news is that you only have to do the math once yearly because your numbers are valid for as long as you are that same age. To make your workouts easier, stay close to the first number above, and to make them harder and increase your fitness level, work closer towards the second number above (B). Note: A certified personal trainer can help you make these numbers more specific for you, but for now this is a good way to set a starting range.

J

JOY

Common question: "Why should I exercise when there's no joy in it?"

In the trilogy of cardiovascular, strength, and flexibility fitness, we often overlook the fact that these are means to an end, and not the ends in themselves. An overall increased quality of life proves to be the best by-product of a fitness program. Indeed, more and more fitness programs and trainers are changing their names to *wellness* programs and *wellness* trainers to amplify the role of well-being. We tend to think of *fitness* as relating to a gym or class, but the term "*wellness*" relates to all aspects of life. When one's body performs efficiently and functionally, allowing one to achieve all daily tasks, one possesses quality of life. From sleep to daily tasks, the truly healthy individual not only boasts contentment, but also joy. Joy is the emotion of happiness mixed with exhilaration.

My medical care practitioner in New York City believes in the power of joy from the integration of a positive mind with a healthy body. Dr. James A. Underberg, MD, Clinical Assistant Professor of Medicine of NYU Medical School, states:

> The first step to a healthy lifestyle is making the decision to pursue one. Encouragement from friends, family or ones own physician should never be overlooked as this source of inspiration. The mental commitment to making a change is the first step to overall health. Mind and body connect in more ways then one. We exercise for many reasons, for weight loss (which reduces the risk of diabetes, hypertension, and cardiovascular disease), for cosmetic reasons, for aerobic reasons (again to benefit the heart) and finally (but perhaps most important) for emotional reasons. Anything we do different today is more than we did the day before, and that is the beginning of a better mind-body connection that leads to overall health and well-being.

This clearly demonstrates how an individual's mental state can affect his or her well-being. With all the talk these days of the mind-body connection, we often overlook a *healthy* mind-body connection. One can be void of sickness but may not necessarily be full of wellness.

Finally, remember endorphins! There is no more natural way to bring JOY in your life than by invoking endorphins when you exercise! These are the wonderful chemicals that increase the more you exercise, regardless of the intensity level of your workout.

Joy can help you feel better about being healthy, about being alive, about having a place on the planet. Joy gives you an amazing feeling which helps you live in the present. When you are conscious of feeling joy, you are living truly in the present, for you cannot be joyous of the past or of the future. When you allow yourself to feel joy, know that you are taking time to smell the proverbial roses. You are truly living in the present!

K

KEEPING ON TRACK

Common question: "I started and then stopped for a week. Isn't it just a lost cause?"

The only lost cause is the one that's forgotten, so what matters is that you pick back up the routine that was placed on PAUSE at some point. Keeping on track proves important because we need to make sure that we not only check our goals periodically, but also make sure they remain realistic. It was once said that we should do our part to leave footprints on the sands of time. I say it's even more important to make sure they point in a commendable direction!

To that end, I suggest you keep a simple reward system can help you self-motivate.

On a monthly scale, one way to stay on track is to look at your goals once a month to make sure that your gym routines, personal trainer, meals, and all fitness endeavors all point in that general direction of those very goals. On a weekly scale, you can stay on track of the need for change by asking yourself "What is one new way I can change up my routine this week to achieve my goals?" ON a daily scale, I suggest taking just 60 seconds each day to ask yourself "How will my scheduled activities contribute towards my fitness goals today?" If for some reason you don't have a positive answer, such as "Not much because I'm spending all day sitting on a plane" or "Not much because I have to sit at my desk all day and prepare my taxes with no time for the gym," recognize this with no negative judgments. The aspiration is to be *aware* that your activities on any given day are or are not getting you closer to your goals; the objective is not to judge yourself negatively.

My good friend, teacher, and presenter of QVC Home Shopping Network Sara Kooperman, JD, develops a tally system of rewards with her family, and this may work well for you. For example, every time you do a workout on a treadmill, you can give yourself a tally on a sheet placed on the refrigerator. After you accrue ten tallies, you treat yourself to the movies, a special aromatherapy bath or shower, or special time to peruse a magazine you like. Make some treats related to food, and some not, because behaviors themselves (like going to the movies) should be rewarding, not food.

Tallies could look like the following:

You are not   alone. No
one is alone. You can delegate the
responsibility of keeping on track to others
and share the burden! Be honest with
friends and tell them how they can help
motivate you. Ask someone dependable to
call you at a time when you need to keep
on track (Monday mornings before the
gym, for example). Just ask this person to
remind you of the reasons for doing your
workout as you try to stay on track. Ask
another dependable friend to email or call
you after you workout to inquire about it.
"How was your workout intensity today,"
"Did you give yourself the workout you
needed today," and "I'm so proud of you
for working out when maybe you didn't
feel quite up to it. How do you feel NOW?"
are all valid questions that others can use
to help you stay on track. For anytime
during the month when you find yourself
having difficulty staying on track, ask yet
another friend to call you and encourage
you. Finally, if you attend group fitness
classes, find someone in the classes you
take who lives in your neighborhood who

could either travel to and from the gym with you, meet with you after class for tea, or both. Companionship is another excellent way to keep on track with your goals.

Keeping on track also means making sure that you re-evaluate your needs periodically. In a journal, write the reasons *why* you are exercising, and this can help you stay focused on your feelings and not on the expectations of any 'end' product. The following sample journal entry serves as example:

"Today I walked 20 minutes because I know I was sitting a lot at my desk. I want to walk because I'm trying to start burning fat with cardiovascular exercise and loose some fat. I felt tired and not motivated at the start, but now feel invigorated."

L

LOGGING, LAPSES, & LAUGHTER

Common question: "What happens if
I miss a workout?"

When individuals approach me over
the years to "give them a fitness regime" or
"give them a diet," my response always is
the same. First, I want to ascertain their
seriousness about making change. It tell
them: "Please come to me having written
down what you've eaten in the past few
days before I sit with you to discuss what
you will eat in the coming months."
Invariably, individuals do not follow-
through. They don't realize that, to make
future change, you have to commit to take
responsibility for your program. People
want a magical approach to fitness or
meal planning. If they are not disciplined
enough to provide me an honest written
log of what they've eaten in three days,
how can they suppose to have the
discipline to face a lifelong future of
change?
    "Logging" is the process of keeping a
journal of a specific purpose: thoughts,
emotions, exercise, meals, emails, tasks,
or even a combination of these. The

purpose is twofold. First, having to write a log helps reinforce commitment to other behaviors. Second, having a log to look back upon helps note trends of discipline and adherence over time. When you know you are accountable to write down your exercise on any given day, you may increase your adherence to your personal commitments. Over time, when you (and a fitness or medical professional) read your log, you will see your initial plan and how it blossomed or bombed.

Logging also reveals your regularity, any lapses from training, and genuine commitment. If you are extremely busy and have no time for your exercise plan, or if you have to eat a meal of mostly fried items, you will record this and, over time, the log will help reveal trends in your life. Small lapses are normal. The most important thing to remember about lapses is that there is no overall perfect plan. Remember that there is no real junk food, but there are junk diets and meal plans: what you do over time is what's really important, not at one meal alone or in one exercise session alone.

Small deviations are allowed. All of the elite athletes I've ever trained have admitted to me taking a day off, eating some chocolate, or having a bit of popcorn at a movie. If these momentary lapses work well for them without major changes to their habits or bodies, then let the rest of us less fit people, too, remember that lapses are normal. A lapse that extends over seven days may indeed produce devastating effects to your overall goals, so remember that short lapses are better than longer ones because you can get back on track faster.

The only constant thing in this world is change! There is no such thing as following a fitness or meal plan regimen perfectly. Remembering this will help you ease up on yourself. It's great that there are no "meal" or "fitness" police out there because we can be our own worst critics. Indeed, I've found that most people don't even *begin* any type of fitness program because they consider themselves unworthy or incapable. Furthermore, when we lighten up to our imperfections and even learn to laugh, physiological changes can occur. The benefits of laughter go beyond heart disease. Laughter has been found to decrease tension and reduce pain. It also appears to boost the body's production of infection-fighting antibodies. "Laughter recently got a boost when researchers announced at an American Heart Association meeting last November [2002] that heart-healthy people are more likely to laugh frequently and heartily than those with heart disease," says Nicole Nisly, M.D., UI Hospitals and Clinics Complementary and Alternative Medicine Clinic. (Iowa:

University of Iowa Health Science Relations, September 2003) "They are also more likely to use humor to smooth over difficult situations. Laughter even has the potential to help in the treatment of depression and other emotional illnesses." Remember the last time you had a confrontation or got angry. How could you have turned that into a humorous event and said something witty, imagining that same scene was being acted out in a television sitcom?

So as you keep logging your progress—and even noticing your lapses— try to relax and try not to take any fitness or meal program too seriously because the only reason that angels can fly is because they take themselves so lightly!

Sample Log

date duration	time	food consumed	how much	type of activity

M

MACHINES

Common question: Those machines at the gym intimidate me.

Machines can make our work lives easier. For some readers, there was a time when typewriters were really 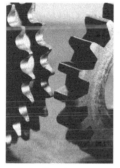 groundbreaking inventions. Then came word processors which revolutionized the typewritten page. Personal Pocket Assistants combined with mobile telephones and cameras are the current craze, which concentrate all of that information into a small, handheld space, and they work quickly and efficiently.

Fitness machines can enhance our fit lifestyles. There are two types: machines which possess researched and true benefits, and machines which dupe people but really hold no true benefit potential. Both types are found both at home and in some fitness facilities.

Machines can assist in all aspects of our fitness trilogy: cardiovascular, strength, or flexibility training.   Large strength training machines can first appear intimidating. These make you stronger because you move heavier weight to work the muscles. Some flexibility-enhancing machines like Pilates machines and sitting-to-stretch machines are a little less common. Still other machines are cardiovascular machines like treadmills, bicycles, and stair-climbing machines. When you sit upright on a bicycle, it's called 'upright,' and if you sit and recline backwards a bit, it's called a 'recumbent' bike. The latter makes cycling easier for the new-to-fit individual because it requires less upper-body strength to sit

The purpose of all of these cardiovascular machines is to help you get closer to your goals in a way that you couldn't do on your own. Cardiovascular machines help you increase your caloric expenditure so you sweat, burn calories, and lose fat. Among the safe and industry-accepted machines, no particular machine is better at helping you burn fat than another, so just choose one that does not intimidate you. The best one for you is the one you are willing to use the longest with the most enjoyment. Try to stay with a cardiovascular machine for a minimum of 12 minutes. If you get bored, move to a different machine. One of the wonderful aspects of machines is variety! Say you want to exercise for 20 minutes.

If you chose 3 different cardiovascular machines, you only need to spend 7 minutes per machine to give yourself the benefits of a great beginning 21-minute cardiovascular regimen! Time really seems to fly when you're only on a machine for 7 minutes!

When approaching a cardiovascular or strength machine in the gym for the first time, ask for assistance. Even the most elite personal trainer herself or himself can find it a bit intimidating when faced with the plethora of controls on a newfangled machine! Most machines now have buttons called "quick start," which help the exerciser bypass the entering of data like age, weight, height, and specific pre-programmed computer workouts. "Quick Starts" allow exercisers to get on a machine, determine his or her timeframe, and get off with results! Remember, too, that you most likely do not need to use machines for hours like some people you'll observe in the gym. Research shows that health benefits occur with an investment of as little as ten minutes! For example, American Council of Sports Medicine (1995) and Reebok University (1999) report that an accumulation of 20-30 minutes of moderate intensity (only between 11-13 on our Intensity Scale described in "I"), equivalent also to 3 sessions of 10 minutes/sessions per day, 4-6 days of the week, will produce health gain benefits.

Be wary of some machines. Of the machines that do not work are the machines that claim to spot reduce (see "S") and also those that stimulate individual muscle sites in the body, usually electrically. There is no proven research that shows that electrical stimulation of the muscles in any area of the body by these machines causes those muscles to contract through their full range of motion in such a way that will make them stronger or more defined. If you shuffle your feet on a carpet with shoes and then touch a metal doorknob, you perhaps will feel a spark, but this doesn't mean that electrical current throughout your body will make your muscles any stronger! The same is true with many gimmick machines on the market you will see. While some are valid home-versions of larger gym machines, others are get-rich quick schemes coming from expensive, but gorgeous, infomercials with false promises.

How do you know when a piece of equipment you see on tv is valid? Ask your gym. Chances are that if a program or piece of equipment is sound for your body, the better fitness facility will have its own version of that very equipment. This is a great rule of thumb.

Other pieces of equipment abound. While they are not machines, these 'fitness toys' also enhance strength, flexibility, and balance: Reebok Core Boards, foam

rollers, inflatable balls, half ball BOSU®
trainers, stability disks, weighted balls
called "medicine" balls. Many consumer
videos are available for using these
products both in gyms and at home.
Because they exist for both home and
gym, they are often valid. Training is key
so you know how to use these objects
properly.

N

NEW

Common question: "I hate starting to exercise because I always get sore. How do I eliminate that part?"

There are two scientific principles that summarize what happens to muscles when you use them, the G.A.S. and S.A.I.D. principles. I will make it easy for you by telling you how I learned them. G.A.S. stands for the "General Adaptation Syndrome," while the S.A.I.D. stands for "Specific Adaptation to Imposed Demands." Together, they both mean that your muscles are very intelligent at becoming efficient when being used. When you first try something new, like walking, rock climbing, or pushing a new vacuum cleaner in the house, the next day you may feel something different in the body. Soreness isn't always bad: it means that you've given something new for the muscles to do. Soreness is feeling a body area in a new way, and it is dull. Pain, however, is sharp, and needs to be attended to by a medical care practitioner.
    If you keep walking, rock climbing, or pushing that new vacuum cleaner *in the same way* (same amount of time, same intensity, same length), shortly you will

notice that you won't get sore because your muscles "learn" how to adapt very well to that *specific* equipment in that *specific* place in the house. It's no wonder that, in fitness, we call this the principle of *specificity*.

Muscles should adapt because life is more functional and easier when we're not sore after every activity. However, if muscles don't get challenged sometimes with new patterns of movement, they never reach new levels of fitness. When this happens, muscles that aren't challenged can become weak and then consequently set you up for injury. (See "Quitting"). The balance between old and new patterns for the muscles is what makes fitness fun and exciting!

And here's the crux of why so many individuals fall off of the wagon with fitness: in this initial phase of soreness, they get frustrated and believe that fitness always will make them feel discomfort like this. This is not so, however! Shortly (between one to two weeks), the soreness disappears, leaving just the great benefits of stronger muscles! The first message of this section is this: if we remember that the soreness is temporary, then we can stay with our fitness plans knowing that the *permanent* benefits will outweigh any *temporary* discomfort. Being a bit *sore* is quite different from being *injured*. When you feel your muscles with a dull ache, this can be an indicator that you have accomplished the task of training your muscles in a new way!

Now you understand the good news about muscle soreness: it exists whenever we give a new pattern of movement to the muscles. Remember that this new pattern can be as subtle as changing from walking on a treadmill in the perfect environment of a gym to the real outside terrain, facing such things as hills and different walking surfaces. Your ankles work differently between a treadmill and the soft sand at a beach, for example.

The second message of this section is this: since we know that muscles adapt quickly to become efficient, diminishing the soreness over time, it behooves us to change up the way we work our muscles from time to time in order to challenge them differently. While a bicep in your upper arm is always a bicep regardless of what it lifts, changing the way you use the bicep (changing the angles, weight, and speed involved, for example) affect the way the bicep will get trained. For example, if you carry home light bags of groceries from the grocery store daily, you will feel sore the day after you carry home a log of wood for the first time because your muscles aren't yet adapted to the heavier weight. The more *new* changes you give a muscle or group of muscles, the more you are exploring the full potential of all of the muscles within you.

Change doesn't need to apply just to your fitness life. Think about making small changes to routine just to spice things up a bit and wake up the body from sleeping in the ordinary run of things. Even if you decide to try to brush your teeth with the hand you normally don't use, that's still change! If you decide catch up on emails before television instead of after, this is also an example of a change.

Regarding changing up your physical exercise routine, remember that a personal trainer is one of your best resources when deciding how to add these small changes of varied angles, weight, and speed to your routine.

O

OBSERVATION

Common question: "Why do fitness people always just look so good?

    A good section of improving your fitness deals with becoming aware of your own body in space and time. As you read through the following questions, know that the purpose is not to judge the answers, only to become *aware* via the questions. Just being able to answer is the purpose. If you want to change the way you answer the questions, address those issues with your personal trainer. People involved in fitness do not possess perfect bodies or perfect eating plans, but they do possess an acute awareness of their lifestyles so that the have an *overall* awareness of themselves, from posture, to how much movement they give themselves in any given day, to what they eat.

    The technical term for this skill of starting to understand your body better is called **kinesthetic awareness**. Practice becoming more aware of the following parts of your involvement in wellness.

Sleeping:
When you sleep, try to notice the position of your joints: ankles, knees, hips, elbows, and shoulders. Are they bent for most of the night? Do you sleep face up or down more? Are the sides of your body symmetrical? Do they change often during the night? Do you often wake up to urinate? Do you often wake up? Do you remember your dreams? Do you fall asleep within five minutes of your head's contact with the pillow, or does it take you longer to fall asleep? Do you awaken feeling tired or rested?

Awaking:
Do you awaken naturally without an alarm clock? Do you always need an alarm clock? How do you feel when you awaken? Do you jump out of bed or stretch your muscles in some way? When you sit on the edge of your bed before contacting the floor, how do you feel? How do your joints feel: ankles, knees, hips, elbows, and shoulders?

Working:
Do you spend most of the time sitting with the hips and knees bent, as in a sitting position? Does your posture lose

alignment by hunching forward at a computer screen, kitchen counter, television, or desk? Does your posture lose alignment by bending to the side or backwards when you rest? How much of your day do you spend sitting (car, couch, table, desk) and how much are you actually moving through space and time (walking, climbing stairs, running, bending, exercising).

Traveling
In what position do you spend most of your time? Are you sitting with the hips and knees bent? How much water do you consume if you had to divide it into flight hours?

Feelings and Food:
Are you able to recognize hunger? Do you wait until you are hungry to eat? Do you always eat when you are hungry? Do you eat when stressed? Do you snack? Do you eat one, two, or three big meals, or do you have many frequent small meals? Do you have a typical, predictable meal plan? Do you snack on predictable foods? Do you ever use words like "good" and "bad" in relation to your behavior with food? Do you sometimes want to skip a meal because of eating a particularly large one (like "Thanksgiving dinner") the day before? Do you chew your food carefully, or gulp it down, sometimes with conversation as you eat fast?

P

PROPRIOCEPTION: STABILITY AND MOBILITY

Common question: "Everyone seems to talk about balance training these days. I wasn't born with good balance, so what's the point?"

Proprioception is a fitness word that means "the ability to control where you are in space and time at any moment." A simplified word for proprioception is "balance." In your body there are muscles that have specific names, and some of these fit into the category of "proprioceptors." These muscles not only contract for functions on the joints, but also have functions to help you balance. The muscles up the front of the lower leg are the anterior tibialis muscles. They run

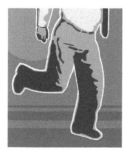

along the shin bone and are responsible for dorsiflexing (raising) your toes up to the sky when you stand as if you were going to walk on your heels. Whenever you stand on one leg, these muscles on your support foot don't contract and bring the ankle up towards the sky (because you'd fall over if they did) but instead contract with no movement (called an "isometric" contraction) to stabilize almost everything: your ankle, knee, hips, and the entire upper torso in proper balance. Thank goodness for these proprioceptor muscles of the ankles and arms that contract so that we keep our balance!

Nobody is born with awesome balance: balance is something you train. If this were not the case, then we would be born walking on 2 legs instead of having first to crawl, or we would be able to ride a bike on 2 wheels instead of having to learn balance with the help of 4 in the beginning.

Why is proprioception (balance) training so important then? Matt Lauer of the NBC Today Show in 2002 reported in November that the number one cause of death of Americans in 2000 was death by falls and related accidents. The International Council on Active Aging reports (http://www.icaa.cc/ newsletters2003/newsletter/Vol3_Issue30 .htm) that falls mark the beginning of the end for many individuals over fifty as the number of documented falls increases yearly. In 2006, the New York City Transit Authority published that in subways 74% of its 2005 accidents occurred because of "falls, slips, and trips" (www.mta.info/reports). If people learn to train both their stability and mobility together, called "balance," then they help minimize these risks.

How do you train both stability and mobility? Think of walking across a hotel lobby that has different surfaces. You walk with speed and confidence when there's thick carpet, but react differently as soon as the carpet yields way to marble floor, and then react yet again when you see someone mopping that wet marble. When you are proprioceptive, you are able to walk on all surfaces without falling because your muscles talk to each other, communicate with each other, and, ultimately work with each other so your body can react so you don't fall down. This means you are stable (because you don't fall) and mobile (because you continue walking along). As a Reebok University Master Trainer, I enjoy helping others learn about these two fundamental concepts of stability and mobility as they relate to proprioception.

Getting all of the muscles to work together is of utmost importance in training today. Traditionally, we went to the gym and worked from machine to machine, asking the body to train only one body part at a time in *isolation*. Some machine manufacturers make us quite comfortable in those machines by giving us padded seats, headrests, and even seatbelts to strap ourselves into to be sure that nothing else moves but that one muscle. The irony remains that, as soon as we unlatch ourselves from those machines and walk away, the mere act of walking towards daily life recruits many different types of muscles all over the body working in an *integrated* fashion! To be sure, machine training has a place in training, including rehabilitation, muscular strength, and hypertrophy (making muscles big), but it seems to me that, since the body is made to function as an integrated unit, we should train the body as an integrated unit, and research across the globe supports this.

Finally, if we spend at least some of our time training the body in an integrated format, we save time by training more body parts simultaneously! Remember, then, to address balance with your personal trainer. If you don't have the opportunity to work individually, learn some great exercises with or without equipment that you could do at home. Check out www.power-systems.com for unique programs that enhance your balance.

TRY THIS:

And in the meantime, stand on one leg. Nothing is a great test of your ability to work all of the muscles down one side of your body like standing on one leg. Hold onto a chair or table if you must in the beginning, but gradually progress to being able to stand on one leg for longer periods of time, with your eyes closed, and even doing a few mini single-leg squats in which you bend the supporting knee just an inch or so, then return to neutral.

Q

QUITTING

Common question: "Every time I start to exercise, I always fizzle out. How do you guarantee I won't this time?"

I've heard that most people that fall off of diets or exercise programs quit because they don't have time or money to keep going. Do you believe those 2 excuses? While it may be valid, appropriate exercise doesn't have to cost much or even take up a lot of time. Remember the research we review in section "M" proving that an accumulation of 30 minutes of moderate intensity (equivalent also to 3 sessions of 10 minutes/sessions per day), 4-6 days of the week, will produce health gain benefits. That's amazing! It also negates our excuse that we cannot find enough time in our days to exercise, because everyone has time to make ten minute sessions! Furthermore, it doesn't have to take an investment of anything more than a good pair of Reebok walking shoes to get out of the house and into a better quality of life through walking.

Why else would people stop exercising, then? Muscular soreness is one reason. We began to discuss this in "N." When muscles that are used to sitting and walking do some different activity (like gardening, kayaking, or snowboarding for the first time), they get sore. This is called Delayed Onset Muscle Soreness, or DOMS. We can feel DOMS anywhere from 12-48 hours after working out, and it slowly diminishes with hydration, stretching, and time. DOMS doesn't mean we've done anything detrimental to our body when it feels like discomfort; it means we've asked the muscle to learn something new, and this is positive change. (If there is pain, however, then our body tells us we may need to seek a medical professional!)

People who quit fitness regimes because of soreness forget that, if they continue the same exercise in the same way, DOMS will diminish quickly. The more you train in the same way, the more your muscles face adaptation. Only after we make changes to our routine, which should happen every few weeks, will DOMS reoccur. DOMS is not a lengthy visitor, but is one of the most common reasons why people stop exercising!

Staying motivated to avoid quitting means remembering that soreness isn't permanent, and having a buddy can help. Holding each other accountable to exercise programs can help avoid this phenomenon.

Another reason people quit could be they stop seeing results. At the start of an exercise program, results may surprise you at how quickly they come. Because of adaptation, however, the more you continue to exercise in the *same* way, the body will stop responding quickly. This doesn't mean that you can't do the same workout for years, but it does mean that a time will come where the same routine will not give you any new results. Our bodies need change!

People quit oftentimes about a month into a routine when they stop seeing results with the same intensity as when they first start. Instead of letting this happen to you, just remember to change up your routine often. In other words, when you stop noticing results, it's your body telling you that it's a great time to effect change in the way you train it. Instead of quitting, then, just plan a new course of action for your muscles. Any qualified personal trainer knows this and can assist you in planning this course of action.

Whatever happens, remember that quitting doesn't mean that you are a failure. As many people fall both "on to" and "off of" diets over the course of their lives, the same occurs with fitness routines. If you do stop working out for a time, this doesn't mean that you have quit permanently! There is no rule that says you cannot begin again after you have tried with unsuccessful results. In the truest sense of the word, quitting something is to try only once and never entertain the possibility of doing something similar again.

Find what works for you, what gives you results, and what gives you genuinely the most amount of enjoyment, and you won't be a quitter in fitness.

R

RESISTANCE & STRENGTH TRAINING

Common question from females: "I don't want to get big bodybuilder muscles so I don't lift weights. Is there another way to get stronger without showing muscles?"

Muscles need to be worked or else they get smaller from disuse, called atrophy (pronounced /á-tro-fee/). When you work a muscle so that it can move a heavier object one or two times, that's called *muscular strength*. The purpose of muscular **strength** is to be able to do some tasks everyday, like carrying a heavy load of laundry down the hall or pulling out the washing machine because something fell behind it. When you work a muscle so that it can move a lighter object many times in a repeated fashion, that's called *muscular endurance*. Even walking is an example of muscular endurance, because you are using your muscles repeatedly with a light load. The purpose of muscular **endurance** is to be able to do everyday task more efficiently without injury, like opening car doors, walking, and taking the stairs.

As you can guess, both muscular strength and endurance are important! Muscles should be trained two different ways: using heavier weights for fewer repetitions (training **strength**) and using lighter weights for more repetitions (training **endurance**). Consult with your certified personal trainer for the best combination based on your individual goals and needs. Contrary to popular opinion, however, females who lift the right amount of weight will not "bulk up" when they do 3 sets of 8 to 10 repetitions of any given exercise.

Many often ask what the best order for strength and cardiovascular training is. While many visit the gym and practice cardiovascular exercise first as warm-up activity before continuing with weight training, current research actually also supports the reverse. Try warming-up with light weights or some lighter cardiovascular activity such as treadmill walking at a moderate pace, then strength training, followed by cardiovascular endurance last. During the strength training, the body produces a chemical called lactate (the "burn" you feel in the muscles) which turns into pyruvate, a chemical that stays in the body and actually turns into a form of fuel for the cardiovascular activity. This can give you more benefits from the cardiovascular aerobic portion of the workout! To be sure, you don't have to train both cardiovascular and strength on the same day, and starting with cardiovascular work is also good, but this latest research reveals starting with weights first is also a great way to go (Kravitz, L. & Dalleck, L.C. (2002). Physiological factors limiting endurance exercise capacity. IDEA Health & Fitness Source, 20(4), 40-49.).

S

SPOT REDUCING

Common question: Individuals approach me and grab a few inches of their waistline, asking "What's the best exercise to reduce this part?" "What exercise is best for the love handles?"

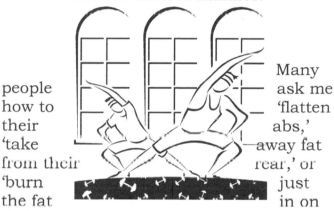

people how to their 'take from their 'burn the fat Many ask me 'flatten abs,' away fat rear,' or just in on their thighs.' The truth is that—apart from surgery such as liposuction-- there is no such thing as fitness spot reducing because the body either puts on fat or burns fat: from all over the landscape. As long as we're alive, we are 'aerobic,' which means breathing and processing oxygen. Those old class terms of "aerobic classes" meant dance and sweat, but now they are aptly named "group fitness classes." "Aerobics" as a term really just means 'processing oxygen.'

Even when we are sleeping, we certainly are 'aerobic' because we are breathing, although we are not doing any particular aerobic exercise. At rest, we burn fat, carbohydrates, and proteins. When we work hard in exercise, we burn more fat, carbohydrates, and proteins. The harder and longer we exercise, the more overall calories we burn, and the good news is that, the more calories we burn, the more we will lose fat from *all* deposits on the body, not just from specific areas. Research tells us that we *burn and lose* fat when we burn more calories than we consume in a typical day. We *store* fat when we consume more calories than we burn in a typical day. Even if we eat 2 boxes of fat free cookies, if we are consuming more calories than the body needs or burns in a day, those fat free cookies will be still be stored as fat because there's no other use for them in the body.

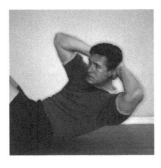

When people ask me to show them exercises for toning muscles of specific body parts, like side-lying leg lifts to reduce the are around the glutes or crunches to reduce abdominal fat, for example, I explain that any exercise most definitely *will* work the muscles in that area, but it will not burn the fat in that area. The muscles will get stronger and more toned. Without cardiovascular activity, however, we will be left with stronger muscles and the same fat deposits in those areas!

We must remember here our trilogy of fitness: to be completely healthy, we should address overall strength, cardiovascular work, and muscular flexibility. Those side-lying leg lifts will work the strength of those muscles, but not give them any cardiovascular benefit of fat burning. Let's remember that a pound of muscle and a pound of fat weigh the same (it's still a pound), but muscle (created by toning) is more *dense* than fat. The American Heart Association tells us that we must work on minimizing fat deposits and maximizing muscular strength to be functional and reduce risk factors.

The answer, then, is to do cardiovascular exercise to burn the fat all over the body, including the cellulite in the area where the leg meets the hip, plus doing strength and endurance types of exercises like those side-lying leg lifts, because they will tone the muscle where the leg meets the hip (called the gluteus medius). Not only will you reduce the amount of fat by burning it off, but also you will have toned muscles and legs in that area to boot!

After people realize that spot reducing won't decrease body fat in a specific area, but that cardiovascular exercise will decrease fat stores throughout the body, the next question is "What does research say about the best form of cardiovascular exercise?" Petra Kolber, former IDEA Instructor of the Year Award Winner, says "the answer is whatever mode of exercise you genuinely like doing is best." As we saw in the Introduction, when *you* make the choice of a form of sweating that helps you work your cardiovascular system in an intense way, you are more likely to stay in that exercise regime for the long run, avoid dropping out, and increase your intensity investment. Results, then, will be favorable.

T

TRILOGY OF FITNESS

Common question: "Can you just tell me
what I have to do to be as fit as you?"

All preceding sections allude to the
trilogy of fitness. Fitness is a three-part
triangle consisting of flexibility,
cardiovascular work, and strength.
Sometimes people spend great deals of
time on one of the three. What's more, the
ironic aspect of fitness trilogies is that I've
found that clients tend to spend the most
amount of time working on their strongest
corner of the three in the trilogy of fitness.
Hercules, for example, probably doesn't
want to spend much time stretching in
yoga class, but developing strength,
instead.

In our "P" section, we discussed
balance as it relates to proprioception.
There are other aspects of balance,
however, like the balance among these
aspects of your fitness trilogy. Please
remember to return here to read this
suggestion: ***always strive for a training
balance among these pinnacles of
fitness***. If you know that flexibility is your
body's weaker link, try to diminish that

weakness by stretching more. You can have a favorite, but overall balance leads to an increased overall quality of life. The more we balance our triangle, the more we can avoid imbalance, injury, and future suffering. Anecdotal information shows that most probably you will injure yourself in your weaker link, not your stronger link. There are no studies that prove that stretching, sweating, and strengthening each day is mandatory. Studies do show, however, how important each of these modes is to stay well.

U

UNDERSTANDING THE INFORMATION OUT THERE

Common questions: "Everybody seems to say something different in fitness so how do I know where to go to get the right answer?" and "When I watch tv infomercials, how do I know if a product or service will work or if it's a waste of money?"

It's hard to understand fitness information based on what's on the television, periodicals, and radio. Almost every day, a different fad diet seems to permeate the market, and so many boast of promises that really are not backed by research. Anyone who has surfed the cable channels quickly becomes confused by the different information given by different infomercials, each promising a fit body faster and better than the first. The American Council on Exercise has become known as the nation's "Workout Watchdog." Over the years, the non-profit organization ACE has commissioned research and testing of exercise products, techniques, and trends in an effort to educate the public. ACE recently prompted the Federal Trade Commission to take action against several companies making false claims on television to protect consumers who have no way of knowing that the claims are false.

Always remember: if there really were an effortless or a quick scheme to dieting or fitness, wouldn't those of us in the fitness profession full-time be aware of it? When you really have concerns about the validity of the claims associated with a product, find out if this information comes from a reputable source by checking www.acefitness.org and www.ideafit.com first. Their websites have "fitness watchdog" sections in which they validate or refute claims of popular products sold on television. *You can find a complete list of valid internet resources under LINKS at my website, findLawrence.com.* I only list products, services, and companies on my website that I believe are ethical and valid.   If you don't have internet access, call ACE in the USA at 800.825.3636 to see if they have any report on any particular specific fitness product in question. You also can ask your currently certified personal trainer. Just because something may be a popular fad does not mean that it works!

Be wary of anyone telling you that he or she has THE ONE FINAL machine, product, pill, or answer to make fitness quick and easy. Fitness isn't a quick fix; it's got to become a lifestyle slowly but surely. If there WERE a magic machine or quick way to achieve wellness, don't you think that all of the healthy athletes, instructors, and personal trainers out there would be using it?

The take-home message here is that there is no quick way to get fit, but fitness routines can be quick! We have seen that spending ten minutes alone on your body is better than nothing at all, that initial soreness will go away, and that little steps towards fitness can yield huge benefits in your body. It's interesting to note that the American College of Sports Medicine and Reebok University reported respectively in 1995 and 1999 that an accumulation of 30 minutes of moderate intensity (RPE 11-13), equivalent also to 3 sessions of 10 minutes/sessions per day, 4-6 days of the week, will produce health gain benefits. Those 30 minutes don't have to be consecutive, so a brisk 10-minute walk done in the morning, repeated at lunch, and repeated at dinner, can produce the same health benefits as doing the 30 minutes consecutively in one bout of exercise!

The key to understanding the contradicting message out there is to find a few key sites and mentors or trainers and stick with them. Remember, if you ever need help finding me to research any important aspect of fitness, you can contact me through my website at findlawrence.com.

V

VITAMINS, MINERALS, & SUPPLEMENTS

Common question: "How do I know if I should take vitamins? Which ones? Can your body absorb vitamins from pills?"

Everyone wants to know which vitamins and minerals to take. Leading personal training organizations believe that the absolute best way to determine what you need is to consult both your medical care practitioner and your Registered Dietitian. You can find a Registered Dietician in your area at www.eatright.org. Your doctor will understand your medical history and any possible drug interactions that may occur in discussing supplementation.

With the exception of some vitamins in the form of oils, vitamins and minerals provide absolutely zero amounts of direct energy, zero amounts of calories, zero amounts of fat, carbohydrate, or protein power. Think of the traditional gas-powered automobile. The most important fuel for the car to run is gasoline. It must be replenished often. During less-often times, the car needs oil and other lubricants so that it can carry out all of its functions, both major and minor. The oil helps the car process and run on the gas, but, no matter how much oil you put into your car, it still cannot run without the appropriate type of gasoline.

Now come back to your body, and follow this analogy. The food you put into your body is like the gasoline, and vitamins and minerals are the oil. To be sure, your body cannot function without its food sources. The vitamins and minerals help the body digest, process, and absorb food as well as carry out hundreds of other daily cellular activities. They are like catalysts that help your body do its other functions, but, alone, they provide no carbohydrate, protein, or fat calories and therefore cannot safely substitute meals.

You ask: "Does my body need supplements if I don't eat healthfully?" The only way to tell for sure is to consult your medical care practitioner and your Registered Dietician. "Is it true that to get all of my vitamins and minerals from natural food I'd have to eat so many more calories than my body needs anyway?" No, because the body needs vitamins and minerals in super-tiny amounts. For example, the body needs about 1000

Recommended Equivalents of Vitamin A (5000 IUs). It sounds like a big number, but one medium carrot contains about 2,500 Recommended Equivalents, which is over twice the minimum you need! So eating just *one* half of a medium carrot already surpasses your need for that day! Most people do not know this and consume far more supplements than they need without consulting their medical advisors first. When people say "I take vitamins because I'd have to eat too many carrots to get enough vitamin A," for example, this just doesn't hold up based on the facts of what the body actually needs. Small amounts of fruits and vegetables contain large doses of vitamins and minerals!

To be sure, some lifestyles like super-active athletic competitors, de-nutritioned youth, and other populations like travelers can benefit from supplements, but they must rely on the close monitoring of their medical care practitioners for types, amounts, and frequency.

Other supplements today attract attention beyond vitamins: steroids, creatine, and caffeine are but a few. Research is still coming in on these drugs, and often gets posted at websites such as www.eatright.org. A word on caffeine: it is a legal stimulant. A stimulant can be a drug, and caffeine is a legal drug. Be careful if you claim that your meal plan is drug free and it contains caffeine: you may be more correct to say that your meal plan is "free of illegal drugs and stimulants." Current research shows that small amounts of caffeine before cardiovascular exercise can help the body to burn more fat (free up more adipose tissue for fuel) during that workout. This is the equivalent of ½ cup of coffee or 1 cup of tea or ½ can of Diet Coke, for example. The danger is that sometimes people get excited at hearing this and consume too much caffeine, which increases the risk of dehydration, emotional dependency, heart irregularities, diarrhea and other serious complications.

Getting vitamins and minerals from food isn't as hard as people think. That said, your medical care practitioner can help you determine if any vitamins or supplements could give you any additional benefit in wellness.

W

WATER

Common question: "How much water should I drink per day? Does coffee count?"

The body contains over 70 percent water, which is more than any of the other macronutrients. In fact, the body needs more water than even carbohydrates, fats, proteins, vitamins, and minerals put together! Instead of wondering how many glasses of water to drink per day, a better rule of thumb is the elimination process itself. Urine should be clear and copious. Frequent urinations during the day can mean proper hydration. The thirst mechanism falls behind the body's need, so when you feel thirsty, know that your body is already heading to a stage that is dehydrated. As long as your urine is clear, you are probably hydrated sufficiently.

Water is best for hydration purposes. In substitution, some liquids are closer to water than others. Coffee, tea, and soda, while containing many other ingredients that often include chemicals, also contain water and *may*

contribute towards the goal of clear urine
if they do not contain much caffeine.
These days in the US an some
other markets, decaffeinated
black, herbal, and green teas
are available, most of which
DO contribute towards water
intake. Caffeine works as a
diuretic on the body and
helps the body eliminate
more liquids than it may if left
to its own natural cycle.
Remember that we achieve our
goal best by drinking pure water. You
want to rehydrate the body, so just
consume that which rehydrates and only
rehydrates! You don't need extra calories
for rehydration! Water is easy for the body
to use; there is no need for the body to
have to separate the water from other
ingredients such as colors, preservatives,
stabilizers, calories, and other additives to
some beverages. Cooler (not ice cold)
water empties faster from the gut than
warmer water, so remember that if you are
exercising at a higher intensity and want
to rehydrate fast!

     Sports drinks aren't best for
hydration unless you are involved in
marathon-like activities over sixty minutes
in duration. Often, individuals in the gym
will work out in a cardiovascular fashion,
sipping on sports drinks. Instead of
rehydrating, what they really are doing is
slowly replacing the calories they are

burning so they will not be losing any fat at all! When exercisers drink electrolyte-carbohydrate replenishing beverages during cardiovascular exercise such as walking on a treadmill, for example, they oftentimes do little more than drink up the calories they are burning, simultaneously! These exercisers, then, will quickly become frustrated and bemused when the scale doesn't show that they are getting as light as they thought. Only when exercising in extremely intense conditions do fitness organizations like ACE and AFAA (Aerobics and Fitness Association of America, www.afaa.com) recommend sports drinks as replacement. ACE recommends everyone to drink eight ounces (one cup) of cool water for every 10-15 minutes of exercise. A safe suggestion is not to wait until you feel thirsty to drink; just make sure you spread out water intake enough during the day so that urine is clear and copious.

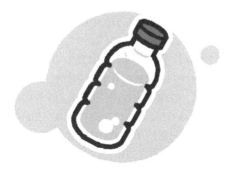

X

XANADU

Common question: "Can you just tell me one ideal plan to get fit?

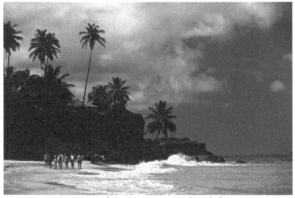

In 1798, the poet Coleridge wrote a wonderful poem entitled "Kubla Khan" in which he speaks of a place of idyllic beauty called "Xanadu." While the poem sounds like a perfect place, and many people want one perfect diet or exercise plan, the truth is that it just doesn't exist. Not every plan works for every person. What's more: the plans that DO work for people don't work for them for their entire lives. Change proves important because we change as well.

I would like to take the reference of Xanadu, however, and extend it to the place inside of us that starts to form when we fuse our mind, body, and spirit, a sort of inner wellness. To be sure, no fitness regime, meal plan, or exercise machine will give you a 'place of idyllic beauty' in and of itself, but the idea of truly embracing health promises more than any one trip to a gym or appointment with a trainer.

Remember that health and fitness benefits are accumulative, which means two things. First, you have to enjoy the good feelings (called "endorphins") that come from exercising after the initial sore stages pass. Second, you have to remember that, the more you do, the more accumulated better health you will have. Far too often, individuals begin exercise regimes, see a quick-start benefit, work through initial soreness, and hit a 'plateau' where they stop seeing additional benefits. Their Xanadu doesn't seem to change anymore. This is the time to put into practice the faith you've developed in yourself and in your workout. Know that little changes will allow you to continue seeking additional rewards. If a workout helps you sleep better or digest food better, realizing that can help you focus on the purpose of fitness in the first place, which is the wellness we have referenced. Fitness may be a healthy body, but, truly, "wellness" is finding that idyllic place of balance among the trilogy of mind, body, breath, and spirit.

Y

YOGA

Common question: "Should I try yoga?"

Yoga comes from the unique language of Sanskrit (from India) and means "putting together" the mind, body, and breath (spirit). In yoga, you move slowly in and out of positions (called "postures" or "asanas") that help take us back to the movements of our animal ancestors, while adding mobility and stability to the spine. When we stand, yoga names come from things like "table" and "mountain," and when we practice yoga on the floor, the names come from animals. There are many types of yoga with many aspects of practice involved, so it's best not to say we 'do' yoga. Instead, we 'practice yoga postures." Take different styles of classes before deciding if something is or isn't right for you. There are many different approaches!

The best way to practice yoga is to get an excellent book and video and read about it first, and then try it slowly. If you want to take a class, find a certified instructor by asking around, searching the internet, and by taking at least three different classes with different instructors before settling into one program. As of this printing, there are no international government standards for yoga instructors, so the safest way to make sure yoga improves your life is to move cautiously as you find an instructor, much in the same way as you find your personal trainer. It's a great idea to use instructors who belong to the Yoga Alliance (yogaalliance.org). If you are new to fitness and to yoga, you may wish to avoid class names such as "power yoga" and "ashtanga," and search out "gentle yoga" and "restorative yoga" because the former tend to be much more intense than the latter.

When you practice yoga, it helps clear the mind because you concentrate on connecting the mind with the body's precise positions to be like things or animals, and then you breathe deeply and completely through the nose. 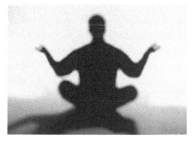 Perhaps more than in any other fitness form, yoga practices careful attention to breathing at all times, called pranayama. For more on breathing, see "B". Other benefits that come from yoga include more of a union among your mind, body, and spirit, an increased body awareness, increased kinesthetic awareness, and improvements in your overall balance (called "proprioception"), mobility, stability, muscular flexibility, and muscular strength, and relaxation & concentration, overall well-being & health.

Z

ZEN

Common question: "What's all this mind-body stuff about anyway?"

Understanding what "zen" is, and adding it to your life in little stages, can improve the quality of your life by drastically reducing stress. Most simply, the concept of "zen" comes from Asian countries and connotes a state of mind in which the body is meditative, free from stress, centered yet directed, and at one with the universe. Although the concept is simple, there is no simple way to define zen, and this is the great paradox of zen.

Zen definitely occurs when one is conscious of being truly present, concentrating on neither the past nor future. This keeps us in the present and helps us avoid anger and fear. You can be angry about the past or fearful of the future, but concentrating on the present help you limit those two emotions and find zen in the present. Zen masters with whom I studied in the kingdom of Bhutan call this feeling "one pointedness" because you direct your attention entirely on the present moment, and usually on only one *aspect* of the present moment at that.

For example, if you sit comfortably, close your eyes, and think just about the quality of your breath in (the inhalation phase) and breath out (the exhalation phase), you may just be thinking about your breathing. Do this long enough, however, and you may find a growing sense of peace, which could be one aspect of feeling zen. When experiencing 'zen,' there is no conscious awareness of social pressure or problems. The relaxation response of the body takes hold and physical changes emerge from what began in the mind. Consequently, as your pulse rate lowers and the body reduces its amounts of stress, many other benefits occur, including reducing risk for heart disease, sleeping better, digesting better, breathing better, and concentrating in a more direct fashion. When the body is at stress, the hormone *cortisol* is produced. Cortisol can lead to obesity, insomnia, and other negative issues. The more you relax and experience zen, the less cortisol your body may produce!

Research tells us more and more that mind-body fitness possesses greater benefits than traditional Western fitness alone because it fuses the trilogy of the brain, body, and breath. When we train all three of these components, our training is more complete and mindful. I define "mindfulness" as the ability *to add careful concentration to whatever you are doing in present time for a deeper awareness.* Adding mindfulness means adding the Eastern philosophy of "zen" to training. The connotation of "zen" not only includes that which promotes concentration, but its connotation also implies aspects of yoga, Pilates, T'ai Chi Chu'an, Feldenkrais, Alexander Techniques, (Guided) Meditation, and other mind-body forms of exercise. Dr. Austin's book *Zen and the Brain* describes in great detail the physiological benefits of sitting in a quiet spot and meditating. He tells us all of the following decrease when we sit quietly and meditate or pray: blood pressure, cortisol, breathing rate, muscular contractions, and perspiration.

Most importantly, the body's self-healing system turns on and activates. This is called the parasympathetic nervous system. When you have a cold or the flu, you feel like lying around and resting or sleeping. This is the body's communication to you that it needs you to decrease other functions so that it can use all of its energy to heal itself. The same thing happens during sections of mind-body exercise like yoga or Pilates or meditation or deep breathing: your body's parasympathetic healing system turns on!

You can add concepts of "zen" to your life in any area you plan to be for five minutes or more by:

*lighting aromatherapy candles so you look at them and concentrate on present-mindedness. Look at the candle and just blink when you need to, noting your feelings. Notice if the pleasant smell helps you deepen your breathing.

*adding any type of relaxing music to your background when you can close your eyes and just concentrate on it

*adding a running water fountain fixture in your vicinity so you can concentrate for a few minutes at a time to the tranquil sounds when you are consciously mindful, and let your subconscious reap the same rewards when you cannot.

*sitting in a quiet area and concentrating on your breathing

*playing softly some inspirational, instrumental music to deepen your mind-body awareness sense.

Now that we've explored the word "zen," your assignment is to find it. Not only when thinking about zen, but I invite you to find it when you are paying attending to any of the concepts in this alphabet guide to wellness. Truly, zen can help you achieve an increased quality of life, regardless if you are at work or play or rest. Adding zen to my life is my new spin, as Mary Poppins sings to the children in Broadway musical:

"If you reach for the stars, all you get are the stars, but I've got a whole new spin. If you reach for the heavens, you get the stars thrown in!" –*"Anything Can Happen"*

WORKS CITED & SUGGESTED READING

Blievernicht, John. "Balance Training." IDEA Personal Trainer. September, 1998.

Brooks, Douglas, MS, and Brooks, Candice Coopeland. "Integrated BOSU® Balance Training: A Programming Guide for Fitness and Health Professionals." DW Fitness, 2002.

Brooks, Douglas. *Effective Strength Training: Analysis and Technique for the Upper Body, Lower Body, and Trunk Exercises*. CA: Moves International Fitness, 2001.

Brownstein B, Bronner, S: "Evaluation Treatment and Outcomes Functional Movement in Orthopedic and Sports Physical Therapy." New York, NY: Churchill Livingstone, Inc., 1997.

Hall, CM, et al.: "Therapeutic Exerciser: Moving Toward Function." New York City: NY: Lippincott Williams & Wilkins, 1999.

Komi, PV, editor. *Strength and Power in Sport*. IL: Human Kinetics Publishers, 1992.

Laskowski, Edward, et. al. "Refining Rehabilitation with Proprioceptive Training." *Physician and Sports Medicine*: October, Vol 25, No. 10: (89-102).

McGill, S. M. "Low-Back Stability: From Formal Description to Issues for Performance and Rehabilitation." *Exercise and Sports Sciences Reviews*, Vol 29, No. 1: (26-31).

Norkin, CC, Levangie, PK: "Joint Structure & Function, 2nd Edition. Philadelphia, PA: FA, Davis Company, 1992.

Reebok Core Professional Training Manual, Reebok University, www.reeboku.com

Reebok Final Cuts Professional Training Manual, Reebok University, www.reeboku.com

Westcott, W. "Golf and Strength Training and Compatible Activities." *Strength and Conditioning.* Vol 18, No. 4: (54-56).

Wolf, Chuck. "Moving the Body." *IDEA Personal Trainer*, 2001, June.

ABOUT THE
AUTHOR

Lawrence Biscontini, MA, has made fitness history as a **Mindful Movement Specialist** as the first recipient of multiple awards from ACE, IDEA & Inner IDEA, Can Fit Pro, and ECA since 2002, currently serving as **Senior VIP Consultant for the American Council on Exercise** (ACE) and **Power Music**®. He creates group fitness and personal training **programming** on an international level for clubs and spas, including Equinox, 24 Hour Fitness, Gold's Gym International, Bally, and Golden Door Spas, where his creations received the **Conde Nast Traveler Awards'** tenth place in the world for innovative spa programming. Lawrence has been **Spa Consultant and Trainer** for leading international spas in Europe, Asia, and the USA. As **Nutritional Counselor,** Lawrence has created complete nutritional menus for spas from Manhattan to Mykonos. Lawrence as **Movement Specialist** enjoys celebrity clients like cast members of ABC TV's soap opera "General Hospital," and appears on news (CNN Headline News) and television ("LIVE! With Regis and Kelly"). He is a **Registered Yoga Alliance Teacher**, an **AFAA Certification Specialist** and **Contributing Author** to industry magazines like AFAA's American Fitness, IDEA's Fitness Journal, and Spa Asia. His **affiliations** include FG2000, BOSU, Beaming, Bender Ball, G Series Fit Gatorade, Gliding, and Savvier. His **books** include the most recent *Musings & Meals*, and *Cream Rises: Excellence in Private & Group Education*. A percentage of all of his website sales goes to his charities of choice, and to inspire career wellness development, he has instituted several Biscontini Scholarships for the fitness and spa community and **"Yo-Global,"** a program to take yoga to the underprivileged. Find Lawrence at www.findlawrence.com.

In the summer of 2004, Lawrence participated in the Opening Ceremonies of the **Athens 2004 Olympics** with yoga and T'ai Chi. *Fitness Magazine named Lawrence one of the **Top Ten USA Trainers** in 2003 (where he served on their Editorial Advisory Board from 1999 until 2007), and cast members of ABC's "General Hospital" in*

ABC Soaps in Depth magazine named Lawrence "fitness guru," to boot.

When not teaching, Lawrence is author *for such international fitness publications as the Human Kinetics release* **Early Morning Cardio Workouts** *with June Kahn, AFAA's Theory and Practice industry standard textbook, and he contributes regularly to ACE Faculty News, AKWA Newsletter Magazine, AsiaFit, SELF magazine, among others. Lawrence's other books include* **The One-Percent Factor: An Eccentric Unicorn's Approach to Touring and Traveling,** *and two fitness yoga texts with eight accompanying videos: Yoga Fundamentals I and II: A Fitness Approach, and Qi Gong and T'ai Chi Fundamentals (available through* **www.scwfitness.com**). *On an international scale, Lawrence serves on both* **IDEA Group Fitness & Steering Committees, Fitness Advisory Board for Fitness Magazine,** *and* **Faculty Advisory Board for the American Council on Exercise.** *For the fitness and consumer market, Lawrence appears in over 40 internationally-sold fitness* **videos** *and* **DVDs.**

Lawrence continues to inspire the world to fitness via various modalities. *First, his company,* **FG2000,** *is a group of leading continuing education providers who offer accredited training at an international level in a variety of languages with a concentration on developing countries who otherwise would not be able to afford this training. For up-and-coming instructors, Lawrence established the* **Biscontini Scholarships** *to offer the opportunity for a promising instructor or personal trainer to attend the* **International World Fitness IDEA convention** *on the west coast USA or the* **SCW** *and* **East Coast Alliance** *events on the east coast, yearly. He also began a* **NOTICE M.E.! program** *through which he helps empower instructors who have innovative ideas in the fitness industry.*

Lawrence's mind-body study *is extensive: with dual Master's Degrees in Spanish Literature & Translation and Education, and a minor in theology, he has studied yoga in India (2006) and in the USA: at Kripalu Center in New York state with yogis from India, under Sri K. Pattabhi Jois (Ashtanga, India), Tias Little, Rodney Yee, Shiva Rea, Donna Rubin (Bikram, NYC), and Molly Fox. Lawrence* *also has studied T'ai Chi under David Dorian-Ross, and Pilates under Lolita San Miguel (student to Joseph Pilates), June Kahn, Moira Stott, and Elizabeth Larkham, Elizabeth Giles. Lawrence studies Feldenkrais under John Link in NYC.*

Lawrence seeks community involvement via fitness. *His company FG2000 takes premier fitness programming to developing countries with a non-for-profit mission, not to make money but to provide education. He founded a T'ai Chi Wellness group in Puerto Rico at a local church community, and taught yoga to incarcerated teens in the Centro de Detención on the island. At the many IDEA Conventions, Lawrence helped raise over thousands yearly for the National Aids Fund at charity workouts, teaching both yoga and T'ai chi to fitness enthusiasts with friend Constance Towers from ABC's **General Hospital**. His cause of choice in the USA is to help the **Sisters of Saint Joseph Villa** based in Philadelphia, a retirement community where both Catholic religious sisters and lay community members alike find care in a wonderful place to live when forced due to health reasons from an active life of nonstop service to others. In the spring of 2004, Lawrence brought fitness professionals together for the plight of New York City animals for the **Broadway Barks Foundation** begun by friend Bernadette Peters. Lawrence served on the board for **Immunocise** in Dallas, Texas, and other organizations that use fitness to help those challenged in some way by HIV and AIDS. He has volunteered for **Workout for Hope**, and was the chief catalyst for Puerto Rico celebrating its first annual Workout for Hope in '98. In 2001, Lawrence initiated a "Fitness Unites" marathon in Puerto Rico to raise money for the **September 11th Fund**.*

Lawrence *teaches in English, Spanish, Italian, and Greek, and is a resident of the world. **Click here to download Lawrence's CV/Resume (PDF)**.*